Praise for Thorns & Roses

"This book gripped me and never let me go until the last page. This is a story of perseverance, faith, hope and love, while enduring unbearable private and physical pain. Cole was able to bring me in and allow me to walk by her side on every page. She tells a story that will leave you in tears, awe, inspired and well informed. She gives the reader a wealth of resources to draw upon, and leaves you with a chapter on lessons learned–full of gems you can apply to daily life no matter what your story may be."

– Peggy Belles, author of *Peace in Pieces*

"Cole very transparently shares her personal life experiences … the pain and sorrow, as well as, the pleasure and joy. She engages within the reader smiles, laughter, pain, tears, empathy, and so much more. I read her book from beginning to end quickly ... couldn't stop ... simply riveted to her story. Whether one's own challenges are similar to or far different than Cole's, her gift of sharing her own story is refreshingly inspiring. Her story makes me want to be a better person: More loving, generous, empathetic, tenacious, giving, and so much more, as a friend, relative, mother, wife, and child of God."

– Betty Barnes

"*Thorns and Roses* is full of the courage, candor, and hope that women fighting sexual pain and dysfunction need to hear from someone who has walked in their shoes. Cole does a masterful job relating the ups and downs of her inspiring journey, while giving women powerful tools and tips for their own journey to healing."

– Emma Strande, DPT

"Cole is open and honest, not only about her physical issues, but also the emotional, spiritual, and relationship roller coaster she and her husband experienced. At first glance, her story offers hope and encouragement to those with sexual pain, but I believe *Thorns and Roses* will be helpful for anyone fighting for their health. Were it not for Cole's tenacity and her willingness to educate herself, she would still be suffering. Healthcare professionals will be challenged to think outside the box and will learn of networks of professionals to which they may refer patients. Cole's writing style is engaging and will hold your attention, even through the clinical portions of the story. Through *Thorns and Roses,* she has "redeemed her story" as she uses the information she learned to reach out and offer hope to those in pain. '*Blessed be the God and Father of our Lord Jesus Christ, the Father of mercies and God of all comfort, who comforts us in all our affliction, so that we may be able to comfort those who are in any affliction, with the comfort with which we ourselves are comforted by God. For as we share abundantly in Christ's sufferings, so through Christ we share abundantly in comfort too.*' 2 Corinthians 1:3-5 (ESV)."

– Mona Turrell, NC, D PSc

"I could not put this book down. Cole writes with a raw passion that is both gripping and intimate–part diary, part thriller. In sharing her intimate journey with others, Cole draws back the curtain on a needlessly private struggle so that others may know they're not alone. But more importantly, she shares how the endless confusion, disappointments and tireless search for answers were equally painful and isolating. And then, once she found her answers and thought life would finally be "normal," she encountered a whole new set of struggles she never anticipated. This book is exhaustively resourceful for anyone suffering with sexual dysfunction, but it's also a beautiful, eloquent tale of a woman's quest for self-discovery and the love of a couple who refuse to give up and stop at nothing to heal their marriage."

- Katy Weber, author of *Worth It*

"From the very beginning, I was gripped by Cole's vulnerable recounting of her journey through tremendous pain and unmatched perseverance. I read the entire book in only two days, staying up late to read because I couldn't put it down. By the end, I felt like I'd made a new friend and rejoiced with her as she at last overcame her battle with pain on so many levels."

- Jennifer Zimmer, author of *30 Days to Thriving*

"Cole holds nothing back in expressing the raw emotions and physical pain she confronted–describing each experience with vivid detail. As a woman who has struggled with sexual pain and chronic vulvar pain, I identified with the author–crying with her pain and rejoicing with her triumphs. *Thorns and Roses* is not just simply Cole's story, she includes a wealth of educational material on the various treatments she tried for her chronic vulvar pain, relevant medical definitions, and resources for additional information. The chapter authored by Dr. Babb is particularly informative. As such, *Thorns and Roses* is a great read for women during all stages of diagnosis and treatment, including those who have not yet received a diagnosis. This book is the whole package rolled up into one and a must-read for anyone who is struggling with vular pain, or anyone who is a loved one of someone struggling with related pain."

– Michelle Living, Director of Support Service
National Vulvodynia Association

Thorns & Roses

THORNS & Roses

A self-help memoir for women with sexual pain

J. Cole

dustjacket

To contact the publisher/author visit www.thornsandroses.us.

ISBN 978-1-947671-22-5

Printed in the United States of America

Scriptures quoted from the English Standard Version of the Bible.

to the 20 million American women who will suffer the physical, mental, emotional, and spiritual effects of sexual pain. May our story give you the strength and courage to persevere. There is hope. There are people who want to help. Please do not give up.

and

to the healthcare providers who understand and dedicate their careers to treating an issue that has been pushed under the rug for far too long–there are not words adequate enough to describe my appreciation for you. So, I simply say, "THANK YOU."

Disclaimer:

This is my personal story. I am not a medical professional. Each person's journey is unique and it is not my intent to diagnose or treat anyone. If you are struggling, please reach out to your primary healthcare provider. Be advised that neither I nor any of the contributing writers can be held responsible for medical decisions made after reading this book.

Contents

Foreword

Women around the world suffer from painful intercourse, but surprisingly few are public about their pain, their attempts at getting treatment, their frustration with lack of proper care, or their joy in becoming pain free. It is a private condition for many, with women often shielding the situation from their loved ones. In *Thorns and Roses* J. Cole literally bares all. As a religious woman married to a good man, she shares her story not seeking the reader's pity nor advice, but hoping to expand the horizons of the reader.

Cole experiences a roller coaster of emotions and physical pain in this recollection of her medical history regarding her sexual function. At times she feels at a loss with herself, with her relationship with her husband, and in her relationship with God. Throughout this book she is open with her thoughts, with her heart, and with her body in order to share her path through the thorns gathering what roses she could find. Now having traversed her path, she hopes her experiences will provide a guide and an inspiration for others–women living with pain, their partners, and their providers.

Thorns and Roses is not only an inspiration, but a resource. It is important that women with sexual pain can relate to others, but it is even more important that they have hope. In this case the hope is provided by Cole in the form of resources.

While sexual pain is devastating, not finding the right support and care is just as devastating. Education is of prime import. The first step to proper treatment is having a diagnosis. Vulvodynia means pain in the vulva … but what is causing the pain? In Cole's case she had multiple issues that occurred after her initial surgery which she recounts in her book—not common, but also not uncommon.

Whether or not you are a woman with pain or her partner, whether or not you are a prescriber or a therapist, whether or not you are religious, whether or not you have children, *Thorns and Roses* will move you and change the way you think about a woman the next time she tells you she has sexual pain.

– "Dr. G."

Irwin Goldstein, MD
Director of Sexual Medicine, Alvarado Hospital
Clinical Professor of Surgery, UCSD
Editor-in-Chief, Sexual Medicine Reviews
Director, San Diego Sexual Medicine

Preface

As I sit here trying to decide what this book is about, I struggle with defining my focus. There are so many avenues it could take–yet the story remains the same. We met, we married, sex was painful, it rocked our world, we sought help, we found none, we had babies, we sought help again, we had more babies, Alan found a book, I called Dr. G, he saved us, we had setbacks, more setbacks, lost each other, lost our minds, lost a child, lost our way, built a house, hated each other, questioned our marriage, became pain-free, started a group, found Dr. Babb, battled to save our marriage, and by the grace of God we're learning to live a good life. So, what's the focus? What's the moral of the story? It is to keep going, don't give up, just when it seems like there is zero hope and zero help left, God will make a way. He will send someone along your path to help guide you. It will be tough. Life is tough. But what is the other option? To give up? To quit? Is that really even an option? I say not.

I wrote those words in a moment of utter desperation–trying to get a grip on the thoughts crashing in my mind like the waves in a roaring sea. Yet, as I near the completion of this book and read back over the words I so quickly threw together, I realize just how true they are regarding the "why" behind sharing our story in such an exposed manner.

Because I am usually the last person to share my deepest thoughts and feelings, it took God more than three years of molding me in preparation for a time when I have no excuse to not share this message.

From the very first moment Dr. Irwin Goldstein suggested I write a book I realized telling our story would make me vulnerable, and that scared me–a lot.

I felt inadequate. Who was I to write a book? I failed so miserably so many times along our journey. I failed to be strong. I failed to trust God. I failed to be me. But as the months passed and the words came together, my fear slowly turned to excitement. Thanks to research pioneer and author Brené Brown, I began to view my feeling of vulnerability as a strength rather than a weakness. In *Daring Greatly*, Brown focuses on the courage that can be found in being vulnerable:

> *"Yes, we are totally exposed when we are vulnerable. Yes, we are in the torture chamber we call uncertainty. And, yes, we're taking a huge emotional risk when we allow ourselves to be vulnerable. But there's no equation where taking risks, braving uncertainty, and opening ourselves up to emotional exposure equals weakness."*[1]

With that in mind, this story is real; it is raw. I did not hold anything back. I want readers to know their physical, mental, and emotional struggles do not mean they are in some way broken. Every single person alive is struggling somehow, somewhere. We may not see it from the outside–most of us are experts at hiding the hard things–but the difficulty is there.

For example, to those observing Alan and me from a distance, our life looks like a tale from a storybook. We had the dream wedding, we have three amazing kids, we built the big house on the hill in the middle of a hundred acres, Alan has a stable job, I get to be a stay-at-home mom, our families both live within 45 minutes of us–we seem to have it all. Honestly, most people who live and work with us daily will never know the trials through which we have been, and that's okay.

However, to those out there in situations similar to ours, this book is for you. You are not alone. You are the reason I stepped far out of my comfort zone and found the strength to be vulnerable. If our story of perseverance can encourage even one couple to keep going–to stay together–then it will all be worth it. Stay strong. There is help. There is hope. There is healing. There is a God who loves you (John 3:16-17, English Standard Version). It may be a rough and rocky road at times, but you have this.

If you are a healthcare provider reading this book, I hope I adequately portray the significant impact that a problem such as sexual pain has, not only on the patient physically, but also mentally and emotionally–as well as, the severe strain it can cause in relationships. Women try to be tough, we try not to complain, but just because we say nothing is wrong, doesn't mean nothing is wrong. I recognize that it is uncomfortable for most professionals to inquire about and discuss a patient's sex life, but I plead with you to grasp the seriousness of sexual dysfunction and at the very least, search out experts in your area to whom you can refer those who come to you seeking help with their issues.

Lastly, to everyone who reads this book, I hope the lesson you take away is the incredible, eye-opening lesson I've learned through these trials: We never truly understand the life another person is living. We cannot walk in their shoes. We cannot know all the reasons behind their actions or reactions. We can, however, choose the way we act and react. So, let us be kind, smile, be patient, speak encouraging words, show mercy, live Matthew 7:12 ... You may not have sexual pain, you may not have a rocky marriage, but we all have something tough in our lives, and I pray to remember that daily.

May God bless you today and every day,

– *J. Cole*

Abbreviations

AASECT - American Association of Sexuality Educators, Counselors and Therapists

Dr. G - Irwin Goldstein, MD

EMDR - Eye Movement Desensitization Reprocessing

ISSWSH - International Society for the Study of Women's Sexual Health

LMFT - Licensed Marriage and Family Therapist

LPC - Licensed Professional Counselor

NP - Nurse Practitioner

NPPVD - Neuroproliferative Provoked Vestibulodynia

NVA - National Vulvodynia Association

PT - Physical Therapy

PTSD - Post Traumatic Stress Disorder

PVD - Provoked Vestibulodynia

SDSM - San Diego Sexual Medicine

VAT - Vestibular Anesthesia Test

SECTION ONE:
to Inform

Compassion is not a relationship between the healer and the wounded. It's a relationship between equals. Only when we know our own darkness well can we be present with the darkness of others. Compassion becomes real when we recognize our shared humanity.

Pema Chödrön

1.

Introduction

We can complain because rose bushes have thorns, or rejoice because thorns have roses.
Unknown

Life is all about perspective. From the moment I decided to write this book, I thought I had the perfect title: *Our Thorn*. At that point, I was still struggling with a recurring cyst, and I thought maybe this was just "our thorn"–our version of the one the apostle Paul writes about in 2 Corinthians 12:7-9a:

> *"So to keep me from becoming conceited ... a thorn was given me in the flesh, a messenger of Satan to harass me, to keep me from becoming conceited. Three times I pleaded with the Lord about this, that it should leave me. But he said to me, 'My grace is sufficient for you, for my power is made perfect in weakness.'"*

Three years later, when I took the leap and enrolled in a book-writing course to bring this work to fruition, I began to rethink my original title. Believing that my sexual pain and its effects on our relationship were "our thorn" was akin to believing in Murphy's Law–the popular adage that "if it can go wrong, it will."

For years I wore the latter as a label, until one day I had an "aha" moment. As I discuss in Chapter 9, the mind has a powerful effect on the body. I realized that as long as I held onto those beliefs, they would undoubtedly remain my reality. So, just as I changed my perspective on life, I also changed the title for this book.

MARRIAGE AND ROSES

Roses–specifically orange ones–are my favorite cut flower. We had loads of them in our wedding. They are my favorite because they smell amazing; their petals are tough enough to stand alone yet stronger together; they grow increasingly stunning as they open with time; and they come in a wide array of shapes, sizes, and colors.

Yet, even in their beauty, roses aren't harmless. Most roses have ruthless thorns meant to protect the plant. It is possible to navigate around those thorns and remain unharmed by them, but one must be diligent and pay careful attention to do so.

Roses also require maintenance. One must choose the proper plant, soil, and site; prepare that site in a manner that will support a healthy plant; monitor the plant for pests; and routinely water, fertilize and prune the plant for optimum growth and flowering.[1]

Isn't marriage much like a rose? It can be a stunning, fragrant piece of heaven on earth.[2] A union in which two strong, committed individuals can come together to create something much more beautiful than if they remained in solitude.

At the same time, marriage also has its thorns. It brings together two fallible people, each with their own unique sets of opinions, beliefs, expectations, and limitations. Without proper handling, each individual can unintentionally harm the other.

Lastly, marriage requires maintenance–intentional, proactive nourishment and protection.

In short, just as roses have thorns, marriages have trials. What a tremendous blessing it is that with a suitable amount of love and commitment, roses and marriages can be two of God's most beautiful creations.

"But he who dares not grasp the thorn
should never crave the rose."
Anne Brontë

MAKE IT YOUR OWN

I did not write this book for sympathy or praise. I would have made us sound a whole lot better had acclamation been my goal. Instead, it is for you, the reader. To give you real-life examples of what to do and what not to do. As a good friend always says, "If you're going to walk through a minefield, follow someone."

The pages that follow are a map of the minefield my husband and I have crossed thus far. We have plenty of battle scars to prove we did not make it through unscathed, but we hope the markers we left on this map aid you in avoiding the dangers we unearthed.

At the same time, this book is yours to read as you want and/or need. If you are preparing for a vestibulectomy and only want to read Chapter 7–it's yours. If you are in the throes of the emotional effects of sexual dysfunction and need to skip to Chapter 9–go for it. By all means, if you want to read every word from cover to cover, I hope you do and I pray you find the words helpful.

POINTS OF EMPHASIS

I could write for days about so many of the topics addressed in this book: Choosing a doctor, healthful eating, reducing stress, lack of desire, benefits of sex, the shame and guilt created by sexual disorders, etc. However, there are great books available that address some of those topics in depth (see the Resources section), so I will spare you a 900-page book. Maybe I will put pen to paper again in the future.

For now, though, as you read through the next 10 chapters, I hope you will keep these overarching principles in mind:

- Sexual pain (or any pain for that matter) may be common, but it is NOT NORMAL. Just like smoke is a sign of fire, pain is a sign of dysfunction.

- You NEED a DIAGNOSIS. We wasted eight years of time, money, frustration, and unnecessary surgery, all with no definitive explanation for my pain. Not cool.

- You must be your OWN ADVOCATE. Do your own research; make your own decisions about your health and how to enhance it. Seek wise counsel, but *you* know *you* best.

- While sex is not the only piece of the intimacy puzzle, it IS a CRUCIAL part of a healthy partnership.[3]

- God is ALWAYS there, willing to help, if we but ASK. I wasn't always certain of that, but through the years I learned to believe Psalm 22:24, "For He has not despised or abhorred the affliction of the afflicted, and He has not hidden his face from him, but has heard, when he cried to Him."

2. Our Fairytale Begins

Once in a while, right in the middle of an ordinary life, love gives us a fairy tale.
Unknown

Like most little girls, I grew up watching fairy tales and dreaming of the day my prince charming would ride in on his gleaming white horse, cradling my lost glass slipper, and sweep me off my feet to live happily ever after on the spacious plains of the Midwest. As I grew older, my favorite movies featured real characters rather than animated, but the romantic plot remained the same: two strangers, surprisingly perfect for each other, meet in a chance encounter, fall in love and live the rest of their lives in peaceful, perfect bliss.

That only happens in the movies you say? I can attest to the fact that it happens in real life as well. The summer between my junior and senior years of college, my prince charming appeared. It would make a great movie, really. It was the third Saturday in June, and though I was exhausted from spending a week as a counselor at a youth church camp, I gladly made the four-hour drive home to attend my roommate's wedding. The following morning, I went to worship with my parents at the congregation where I spent my teen years. I always enjoyed my visits back to that congregation; I loved exchanging smiles and hugs with a Christian family that meant the world to me. Every time I returned, one couple in particular made it a point to find me and ask about college life and classes. This time, though, the husband posed an unexpected question: "Ed (their neighbor and our mutual friend) and I have a guy for you to meet. Is it okay if I give him your number?" To this day I can still hear his voice speaking those words, as I was so surprised by that question. My immediate response was, "Sure!"

After three years of college I'd been on lots of first dates, and many of those were blind dates set up by great friends, but this set-up was different. Not only was the man with whom I was conversing one of great character, the "Ed" he mentioned was a well-respected man I had known from the agricultural education and livestock show circles for as long as I could remember. I was confident that if Les, Mary, and Ed all three approved of someone, I certainly needed to meet him. I quickly found a piece of scrap paper and handed Les my phone number.

That afternoon I returned to Stillwater–my college home. The upcoming week was an especially busy one since I had been gone the previous week. In addition, my 12-year-old niece joined me for the week, as she did regularly. She loved spending time in Stillwater and being my sidekick to internships and activities. Before we knew it, the week was over and it was time to take her home. As she and I began to pack our clothes, my phone rang. It was closest to Brooklyn, so she answered. The next thing I knew she rushed to find me in the next room, eyes lit up, and whispered with excitement, "It's a boy!" I nervously reached for the phone. Little did I know, on the other end of the line was the man who would become my husband in less than 12 months.

BEFORE WE WERE US

I'll throw in a little history here as we set the stage for the rest of this book …

I grew up on a cattle ranch in a tiny Oklahoma town. Born when my sisters were 17 and 20 years old, I was kind of an only child and youngest sibling all wrapped into one. I was blessed to be raised by honest, hard-working, God-fearing parents who taught me to be the same. When I was not mowing or raking hay, stacking round bales, or working cattle, my favorite hobbies included riding horses and showing cattle and pigs. I won a plethora of ribbons in horse shows, was active in the county 4-H club, and later very active in the National FFA Organization. When I transitioned from my local, rural elementary school to the nearest high school, I traded my basketball jersey for a cheerleading uniform–a much better fit for my personality. Post-secondary plans were a given; my mind was set on Oklahoma State University from the time I was born. My college experience in "orange country" was everything I dreamed it would be. I formed lifelong friendships, served in amazing internships, and earned a bachelor of science degree with honors in agricultural communications.

The first 21 years of my life were a piece of cake. Seriously. No drama. No major catastrophes. I was abundantly blessed with family, friends, leaders, coaches, and teachers from whom I learned to be honest, work hard, serve others, love God, and always give my best. They taught me that I could be and do anything I set my mind to. I met little resistance with most things I pursued to that point. That is not to say I didn't have to work hard or never experienced disappointments, but I did learn to expect things to fall my way.

I FOUND HIM WHOM MY SOUL LOVES (Song of Sol. 3:4)

And fall my way they did. On June 28, my prince charming (a.k.a. Alan) pulled up to my parents' house in his white Ford F-150 pickup. Not quite a white horse, but for a country gal it was a close second. That first evening, as he took me to dinner and a movie, he began stealing my heart. The crazy thing was that he did not seem to be the man for whom I thought I was looking. As usual, God had a much better vision of the kind of man I would need. He was not the politician who wanted to live in the big city, nor was he the cowboy who would sweep me off my feet to a 30,000-acre ranch in South Dakota–instead he was a quiet, laid-back, respectful, courteous, kind gentleman whose path crossed mine so many times throughout our lives that only providence kept us from meeting until that summer.

I mean that just as it sounds. Growing up less than 20 miles apart, Alan and I should have known each other. We showed pigs in the same arena as teenagers. I stopped often for mashed potatoes at his family's restaurant when my best friend had braces. I remember his grandmother's name on our church prayer list when she battled cancer. We both attended Oklahoma State for three of the same semesters. We even spent a weekend together at a church retreat where we deloped mutual friends, but never met eachother. Nevertheless, had we met before that summer, we would not have become husband and wife.

Our second date included worship and lunch with my family the following day. Maybe Alan knew that when you marry the person you also marry the family and thought he better check out my "people" before he fell head over heels for me. Really, though, I think he liked me enough he wanted to see me again before I returned to Stillwater. Whatever his motive, I was impressed by his actions. He called that evening to be sure I made it back. He called Monday–and again Tuesday. It had been a long time since I had talked to a guy four days in a row, and I was starting to believe he really did like me. The next weekend, he sealed the deal when he made the two-hour trip to Stillwater to visit me and I anxiously opened my apartment door to see him holding a beautiful bouquet of hand-picked, wild, orange lilies.

As they say, the rest is history. Six short months after we met I went with Alan and his family to ski in Colorado. The second night we were there, Alan took me on a horse-drawn carriage ride through the snow-covered Rockies. When the carriage ride ended, he led me to a picture-perfect campfire where he knelt on one knee and asked me to be his wife. It was literally a storybook scene. Of course, my answer was yes.

AND THEY SHALL BECOME ONE FLESH (Gen. 2:24b)

Like most 20-somethings, I had my wedding planned long before I had a groom: Outdoor, horseback, and OSU orange.

It just so happened Alan's parents had a gorgeous pecan orchard outside their backyard. Two parallel rows of trees formed a natural canopy to shade the 300 white chairs prepared to welcome our guests that mid-June evening. There was one small hiccup: a light rain began to fall about noon on our wedding day and continued through the afternoon. Our decorating crew took shelter in the garage and watched in disappointment as the orange paper lanterns that I had painted so carefully–and they had worked so long to hang–began dropping to the ground one by one. Guests started calling at noon, curious if we were changing locations. I remained the lone, hopeful soul who had no doubt the raindrops would stop falling. By late afternoon, the rain did stop, the clouds dissipated, and the sun returned, leaving just enough time for the ground to dry. The day's moisture ensured the lush grass, green leaves, and lavish landscape looked fresh and crisp. Outdoor. Check.

The second component of my dream wedding trio was to ride into the wedding ceremony on my beloved white(ish) horse, Spook. However, there was a little hitch in the get-along regarding this feat–my white (technically flea-bitten gray) horse hated participating in parades. I was afraid he might think the wedding was a parade, and I might become an unintentional runaway bride. Not something I wanted to chance. Thankfully, my sister's family had a solution. One of their horses was cool as a cucumber in most situations. So, I spent a few days riding their horse through pastures with a bedsheet imitating my wedding dress, dangling across his back and down his legs. I am sure we were a sight to see, but he did great and landed the gig.

Only a handful of people knew how I planned to make my entrance. I am still not sure how my family arrived at Alan's parents' place with a horse in a trailer without raising curiosity, but they succeeded. When it was time, I carefully climbed aboard my trusty mount, gathered the reins, and spread the train of my dress across the horse's back as my devoted father led us around the house to surprise my groom and our guests. Horseback. Check.

I have a funny story regarding our wedding colors. On our way home from the ski-trip, post-engagement, my future mother-in-law about lost it when she asked if I had wedding colors in mind and I quickly answered, "Orange, of course." We were married before orange was in style, but we rocked it. Coincidentally, the tuxedo company started making orange vests that year. Perfect timing. OSU orange. Check.

The rest of our wedding evening was picture-perfect. It was such a dream come true that when they finally scurried us from the reception and we drove away from our magical event, I turned to Alan, with bright-eyes, and asked if we could repeat the wedding all over again. Being a practical, quiet, way-out-of-the-limelight sort of guy, he quickly told me, "No way." Wise man.

Looking back, there are still days I wish so badly that we could recreate the euphoria we felt those first few hours of marriage. Two young souls, high on love, standing before God and our loved ones, committing to each other by exchanging vows–the depths of which we could not begin to comprehend–with a brand-new world before us. It felt incredible.

Little did we know our fairytale was about to have its first reality check.

3

It Glitters, but is it Gold?

Better is an end of a thing than its beginning,
and the patient in spirit is better than
the proud in spirit.
Ecclesiastes 7:8

Our blissful, post-wedding high remained as we arrived at the hotel where we would spend the rest of the night before boarding a 6 a.m. flight to our honeymoon destination: The Canadian Rockies. Everything had moved so quickly from the time we first met, merely 355 days prior. The moment was a bit surreal for both of us as we checked into the hotel as "Mr. and Mrs." As we stood there–me in my white chiffon dress, and Alan in his stark black tuxedo–it was as if we transformed, with the flip of a switch, from 20-something kids into official adults, out on our own, starting our next chapter. The feeling was exhilarating.

We made our way, hand-in-hand, to our hotel room. Upholding tradition, Alan carried me across the "threshold" before he carried our luggage into the room. To keep this PG-ish, I will simply say from that point on, we proceeded to consummate our marriage. A time we had both so anxiously awaited. Life seemed grand.

Only there was a small problem: Life was not grand. Things did not seem to feel quite right. As in, sex was painful and basically impossible. Being inexperienced and somewhat naïve, we both resigned to the assumption that first-time pain was normal and it would take some time for intercourse to feel great. It was probably a stretching or relaxation issue, we thought. Disappointing to say the least, but we knew we had a week-long honeymoon to figure it out.

Neither of us had much to eat that day, so we were extra thankful someone had taken the time to make us a to-go box of the delicious food and cake served during our reception. We enjoyed the fare before showering (where I surprised Alan by nearly passing out from exhaustion), getting a couple hours of sleep, and heading to the airport for our flight to Canada.

Unlike the whirlwind of emotions we experienced on our wedding day, the next day was filled with one over-arching emotion: Blissful freedom. For the first time since we met, we were free from a calendar, a schedule, a to-do-list, a wedding to plan, etc. We were simply able to relax and truly enjoy one another. We spent the afternoon taking in the sights, sounds, and tastes of Calgary. Though we narrowly missed the famous Calgary Stampede (it began two weeks after our visit) we did experience the eager anticipation already in the air.

Our hotel reservation that night was in Calgary. Because we were both running on fumes, we opted to recharge with an early dinner before retreating to our hotel room. Of course, we were also eager to redeem our failed attempt in the "bedroom" the night before. Much to our dismay, the second night was not much better than the first. Intercourse was again painful and awkward. As disheartening as that was, we rolled with it and headed west the next afternoon to beautiful, quaint Banff, Canada. There we enjoyed the hot springs, gondola, and lake. We also found a bottle of massage oil in a downtown boutique to try to spice things up.

From Banff, we spent the week traveling up and then back down the interior of the breath-taking Canadian Rockies. We toured the Colombia Icefield, Jasper and its Spirit Island, and ended our journey at the magnificent Fairmont Chateau Lake Louise. That final destination was the motivation behind the entire trip. When combing through bridal magazines in preparation for our wedding, I ran across an article entitled *Honeymoon in the Canadian Rockies*. The article included an aerial photo of an enchanting hotel that sits at the edge of the picturesque, glacier-fed Lake Louise. Standing beside the lake a few months later with my husband of six short days was absolutely a dream come true.

Our entire honeymoon was unforgettable. In large part because we were blessed to spend our first week as a newlywed couple viewing some of God's most stunning creation. At the same time, we also could not forget the fact that we failed to achieve the amazing sexual experience we both wanted. Despite trying different positions, oils, lubricants, massages, etc., we could not replicate the romantic, intimate, honeymoon sex of which we had dreamed.

THE PUZZLE – DR. #1

As we settled into our new life–one focused on creating a home, finishing college coursework, completing internships, earning an income, and learning to live as husband and wife–I began my quest to find the reason intercourse caused me such pain. I began to backtrack and pull out pieces I thought might be part of the puzzle.

When I was 13, I used a tampon for the first time. It hurt the entire time I wore it. Not knowing any different, I assumed tampons were uncomfortable for everyone, at least in the beginning. I wore them a few more times during my teenage years, but they were always painful. I wondered why in the world anyone in their right mind would tolerate the discomfort caused by tampons.

Until I was 20-something, I did not "provoke" my vagina with anything else. It was around that time I decided to make an appointment for my first gynecological visit with a doctor whom I will call Dr. #1. Even though I arrived at the appointment quite anxious, antipating it would be uncomfortable, I did not expect to feel such a high level of pain during that initial exam. Looking back, I probably should have mentioned the pain to the doctor, but my personality was to be quiet, tough, and just deal with things like pain, so I didn't mention it. After all, I was not expecting my first woman's wellness visit to be a party, so I assumed what I felt was normal and chalked it up as part of the reason every woman talks about the "dreaded" yearly exam. During that exam, Dr. #1 discovered I had a minor vaginal septum (a dividing wall of tissue within the vagina[1]). She said vaginal septums were rare, but it wasn't causing any problems (most of the time I could avoid tampons and I hadn't even met Alan at that point), so I didn't think any more about it.

DR. #2

The spring before our wedding I chose a new, more conveniently located OB/GYN–Dr. #2–and made an appointment to discuss family planning methods (anticipating lots of opportunities for pregnancy, of course). Alan and I both anticipated being married a few years before having children, so Dr. #2 prescribed an oral contraceptive that was popular at the time. As was the case with my first gynecological visit, the entire pelvic exam was painful. However, my goal for the visit was a birth control regimen, and I left having accomplished that goal.

I returned to the doctor for a check-up and contraceptive refill a couple of months after our honeymoon. By that point I knew I had pain with tampons, pain with pelvic exams, and pain with intercourse. Of course, I did not mention any of the three to the doctor. Assertiveness was obviously a weakness at the time. While performing the exam, Dr. #2 discovered a few polyps on my cervix which she removed two months later without complication. Another piece to add to the puzzle, but still no resolution for the pain.

STRUGGLING IN SILENCE

This is probably the best place to add a side note before I get too far into our story. Up to this point, and until about nine years into our marriage, I did not mention a word about the pain or procedures to anyone except Alan. I grew up in a wonderful, Godly family. However, there was very little, if any, dialogue about problems of any kind–and especially not about personal issues. I was born when my mom was 40 years old and my dad 41. As I mentioned in Chapter 2, there was a wide age gap between my sisters and me. My middle sister graduated high school the Friday night before I entered the world on Sunday. She joined our older sister at college a couple of months later. Thus, I was raised like an only child. Later in life we grew closer, but not so close that I would call and discuss something as personal as painful intercourse. That was also not a topic I would ever discuss with our mom. She is a great mother, and I am blessed that she taught me how to serve others, do my best, and believe I could do anything. Nevertheless, we did not develop a relationship that would lend itself to conversations about sexual pain. Right or wrong, I was also uncomfortable mentioning the struggles to my friends.

Sometimes I look back and wonder if I should have handled things differently. Maybe I should have mentioned the pain to someone. Maybe I would have found answers more quickly, or at the very least had more prayers being sent to God on our behalf. I am confident I should have mentioned the pain to Dr. #2. However, the odds that she would have known how to treat me were extremely low and as I've learned through my experiences, all too often most physicians do not take sexual pain seriously.

Hindsight is always 20/20, and puzzles are much easier to assemble when you have a picture to follow. As I look back years later, I am thankful for the grace and strength with which Alan and I quietly played the newlywed cards we were dealt. Our privacy about it all taught us to lean on each other and to lean on God. Vital lessons we both needed to learn and would need to apply in the coming year.

We felt much like King David when he authored the twenty-fifth Psalm.

"Turn to me and be gracious to me,
for I am lonely and afflicted.
The troubles of my heart are enlarged;
bring me out of my distresses.
Consider my affliction and my trouble,
and forgive all my sins."
Psalm 25:16-18

4.

Sending Out an S.O.S.

It is the hard days – the days that challenge you to your very core – that will determine who you are. You will be defined not just by what you achieve, but by how you survive.
Sheryl Sandberg

A little more than a year after our wedding, I decided to see a new OB/GYN, Dr. #3. She came highly recommended by a family friend for her obstetrical skills and knowledge, and for performing ultrasounds at each OB appointment (the standard is to perform a single ultrasound with each pregnancy–usually at the 20-week mark). God directed our steps once again, as the new doctor's diagnostic approach would prove crucial in the upcoming months.

My first appointment with Dr. #3 was routine–the typical yearly exam for a pap smear and physical exam. She entered the room before I undressed to introduce herself and review my history. She was kind and confident. She asked if I had any questions or concerns, so I reluctantly mentioned the pain with intercourse.

Alan and I had been married more than a year at that point, and we basically were never having intercourse since it was still quite painful for me. Even though I could tolerate it, Alan could not stand the thought of hurting me. Thankfully, knowing I was lying in pain was not a turn-on for him.

Dr. #3 proceeded with the exam and "looked" to see what might be wrong. She did not see a physical cause for the pain; however, she did notice the partial vaginal septum that Dr. #1 noticed and theorized that it could be causing my pain. With hopes of resolving the issue, I returned to her office a few days later for an in-office procedure to clip the septum. Unfortunately, the procedure did not alleviate my pain.

Treatment #1: Fail.

Before I left the original visit with Dr. #3, we also discussed birth control options. I had decided after a year on the "pill" that hormonal contraception was not something I wanted to be putting in my body. She asked if we were ready for children, to which I responded with a quick, "No way!" I was certain I could chart my cycle and use a natural family planning method to avoid pregnancy until we were ready. After all, we were having virtually no intercourse anyway, so I assumed that would be a piece of cake. I am not going to put words in her mouth, but I am quite certain my doctor and I didn't share a mutual confidence in my plan. For that reason, I don't think she was surprised when I showed back up to her office a couple of months later pregnant.

OVULATION THEORY

I imagine you are wondering how I became pregnant if intercourse was unbearable. I developed an interesting theory about that in the years that followed. No, not immaculate conception. There is some evidence that decreased pain during ovulation is not uncommon.[1]

One factor for the phenomenon could be the rise and fall of estrogen levels throughout the menstrual cycle. During a typical cycle in pre-menopausal women, the amount of estrogen present in the body can potentially vary from a "normal" low of 27 during the follicular phase to a high of 436 during ovulation (typical serum estrogen levels during menstrual cycle phases: Follicular - 27-123, Ovulation - 96-436, Mid luteal - 49-294)[2]. So, it is possible that the drastically higher levels of estrogen during ovulation produce more "feel good" hormones, which in turn lessen the severity of pain.

In addition, my theory makes common sense, as one of the reasons God created the sexual relationship between husband and wife was for them to procreate. (Genesis 1:27-28)

In the end, my theory may be just that–a theory. Nevertheless, it was a fact that my sexual pain decreased during ovulation. Thus, we had intercourse and created a life. We were shocked, grateful, excited, and anxious all at the same time.

BABY TYLER

I will share a little about that first pregnancy because even though it is not technically related to my physical pain, it did have a major impact on the mental and emotional state of our relationship as spouses and parents.

Remember when I said one of the reasons I chose Dr. #3 was because she performed an ultrasound at each office visit? Well, here's where that comes into play. Alan was with me when we got to see our little "bean" for the first time at my 11-week appointment. While we had not planned to have a child after only 15 months of marriage, we were overjoyed to welcome such a gift from God. We embraced the new life-plan and anxiously awaited the next visit so we could see our baby again–and maybe even learn his or her gender.

The 15-week appointment began much the same as the first. Thankfully Alan was with me once again because as the doctor performed our second ultrasound, she shared with us some devastating news. She observed something abnormal on the previous ultrasound (four weeks prior), but did not want to alarm us at that time. Dr. #3 shared that she'd prayed during those four weeks that she was mistaken about what she saw on the screen, or that something had changed. Unfortunately, the problem she noticed during the first ultrasound was still present. She informed us our baby had major heart defects and prepared us for the worst-case scenario–the reality that there was no way to know how long our baby could survive with the existing problems. I don't have words to accurately describe the wave of emotions that hit Alan and me that cold January day. Nothing in our short lives had prepared us to handle such devastating news about our unborn child.

The next few weeks were full of appointments with pediatric cardiologists, fetal medicine experts, and Dr. #3. It was oddly amazing that they could determine so many things about our baby's heart so early in pregnancy; his heart was smaller than one inch at the time. As the days passed, I felt like I was living in a daze. Strangers would kindly ask about my due date and I would give them a quick answer. It would have been awkward to say what I was really thinking, "Well, he is due July 3, but will probably die before then."

As odd as it sounds, even in the midst of the heartache and uncertainty, we felt God working. Our doctors often spoke the exact words we needed to hear to assure us we were doing everything possible to give our child the best chance to survive and thrive. We continued to pray, although the majority of the time we did not have a clue what to ask of God. I felt selfish praying for our child to live, knowing it was likely his life would be a series of surgeries and pain and fighting. On the other hand, I knew God had the power to heal him completely. As a result, most of my prayers ended something like this: "God, I have no idea what's best for our baby; but You do, and I will have faith that You will work all things for good."

"Likewise the spirit helps us in our weakness.
For we do not know what to pray for
as we ought, but the Spirit himself intercedes for
us with groanings too deep for words.
And He who searches hearts knows what is
the mind of the Spirit, because the Spirit
intercedes for the saints according to the will
of God. And we know that for those who love
God all things work together for good."
Romans 8:26-28a

Amidst the roller coaster of emotions and uncertainty, my wise, older sister–whose first child lived merely one short day–shared a bit of advice she received during their time of infant loss: "However you deal with this, do it together." During times of stress and grief, it is so easy to drift apart as spouses. I am thankful God used my sister to share that wisdom with us, as it played a crucial role in keeping our marriage treading water through some of the most trying times we faced during the next 10 years.

You are probably wondering what happened next with our sweet baby boy. At the 29-week mark I did some traveling for my job in marketing. When I returned to my office mid-week, my co-workers immediately noticed how swollen my body had become and insisted I see my doctor. After performing a battery of tests, Dr. #3 confirmed I had developed pre-eclampsia. Because my blood pressure was crazy high I was put on strict bedrest indefinitely. At the time Alan was working an insane amount of overtime, which added to our stress. By the time he made it home from work the evening of my third day of bedrest, I was extremely ill. In addition, I hadn't felt the baby move all day. I'd been able to fake my way through the day while family members were with me, but when Alan finally got home I fell apart. I knew in my heart that he had passed, but held onto a sliver of hope that maybe he was still with us. When we called Dr. #3 to inform her my blood pressure was up to 160/109, she told us to get to the hospital quickly and she would meet us there.

Shortly after we arrived at the hospital, our doctor confirmed our sweet boy had passed. She quickly prepared me for a C-section and delivered our precious baby just after midnight.

KEEPING THE FAITH

It may sound strange, but as I look back on those days and weeks and months, I can clearly see the way our thoughts, concerns, and prayers were answered by God–in His timing and in His way. We still grieved and questioned the outcome, and get teary-eyed today when we wonder what he would look like, who he would act like, or what he would be doing, but God kept good on His promise to wrap us in His arms and give us the unexplainable peace He promises in Philippians 4:6-7:

"Do not be anxious about anything,
but in everything by prayer and supplication
with thanksgiving let your requests be made

known to God. And the peace of God, which surpasses all understanding, will guard your hearts and your minds in Christ Jesus."

Knowing we have a child in Heaven makes us all the more encouraged to live a life loving God, loving each other, and obeying his commandments (I John 5:1-3) so that we can join him for eternity.

As King David proclaimed after the loss of his child, "While the child was still alive, I fasted and wept, for I said, 'Who knows whether the Lord will be gracious to me, that the child may live?' But now he is dead. Why should I fast? Can I bring him back again? I shall go to him, but he will not return to me." (2 Samuel 12:22-23)

Sweet baby Tyler, it is you we will never forget.
You put a lifetime of love into a single instant.

OUR JOURNEY CONTINUES

From the time we learned about our baby's medical problems until the time he was born, our sexual struggles took a backseat. We busied ourselves with remodeling projects at home, spent hours on end trying to find doctors to help our child, and did the best we could emotionally to handle the heartbreaking journey. The weeks after he was born I spent grieving, recovering from the C-section, preparing to return to my full-time job in marketing, etc. Needless to say, we were both preoccupied.

We celebrated our second wedding anniversary shortly after the baby was born, but felt like we'd already experienced a lifetime worth of sadness heartache.

Once life began to settle down a bit I asked Dr. #3 once again about a solution for my pain. She still couldn't determine a diagnosis so she prescribed a topical estrogen cream. Unfortunately, estrogen was not the cure (which isn't surprising when you read Chapter 6).

Treatment #2: Fail.

You will never guess what happened next … Yep–pregnant, which was utterly exciting and scary all at the same time. Thanks to lots of prayer, ultrasounds, tests, and compassionate doctors who understood our concerns following the previous pregnancy, we were able to control our worry as they assured us our second baby was perfectly healthy. Even with that reassurance, things were a bit intense for those nine months, so once again, our sexual problems were placed on the back burner. The sacrifice and stress all proved worth it when we welcomed our perfectly healthy bundle of boy into our arms.

Topical Estrogen

Topical estrogen, in the form estradiol, is a common first-line treatment for managing vulvar pain. The hope is that the estrogen, applied daily to the vulva/vestibule, will thicken the top layers of skin and insulate the nerve endings to reduce pain signals to the brain. Unlike systemic estrogen replacement - pills or patches, topical estrogen does not increase blood levels of estrogen, and thus is considered very safe. Topical estrogen, and other topical hormones as well, are available in commercial forms (pre-dosed/pre-packaged) or can be individually compounded at a qualified pharmacy by mixing the estradiol into the base most suitable for the patient. Common bases include emollient creams and coconut oil.

Contribution by Jessica Kanwhen, Pharm.D., Bethel Pharmacy

FLORIDA

A few months after our second son was born, we found a ray of hope in a physical therapy clinic that specialized in women's health issues. There was only one problem: The clinic was in Florida and we lived in Oklahoma with a six-month-old. Regardless, we scheduled an appointment and took a "vacation" (that's what we told family, because even then no one knew about our problem).

The owners and staff at the clinic were incredible. For the first time in three and a half years I felt like someone grasped the severity of my dysfunction. Not the physical severity on a scale of 1 to 10, but the severe effect it was having on my relationship with my husband, the severe effect it was beginning to have on my self-esteem, and the severe effect the combination was having on all areas of my life.

Pelvic Rehabilitation

Pelvic rehabilitation is a form of physical therapy that is used to treat several urogenital conditions, including painful intercourse, bowel and bladder incontinence, scar tissue adhesions from Caesarean section or vaginal delivery, endometriosis, pelvic organ prolapse, and vulvo/vestibulodynia. Treatment typically includes internal and/or manual therapy techniques to release trigger points and mobilize scar tissue, exercises to address muscular and fascial restrictions as well as weakness in the hips, low back, and the rest of the body, and treatment to enhance the mobility of the pelvic floor musculature while reducing nerve irritation. Treatments vary depending on the patient's condition, strength, and range of motion, but PT is an excellent way to address these concerns so the patient can return to his or her regular activities without pain or limitation.

Contribution by Megan Warner, PT, DPT, Pelvic Pain PT

After three days of intense pelvic floor rehabilitation, intercourse was much less painful. Nevertheless, when we continued intercourse while I had any level of pain, it felt like the pain increasingly intensified until we stopped. Thankfully, as soon as we stopped, the pain disappeared. In the end, I felt like the treatment was successful in relaxing the targeted muscles and relieving tension, but it did not eliminate the root cause of the pain. Knowing what I know now, I was correct.

Treatment #3: Basically a fail.

OKLAHOMA CITY

Even though our experience at the Florida PT clinic was positive, we returned home disheartened by the fact that we did not discover the *cause* of my pain. So we continued our quest for answers. Much to our surprise, we found a specialist close to home–Dr. #4. He was a urogynecologist in Oklahoma City (about a two-hour drive) who worked in an entire department dedicated to women's pelvic floor disorders. We felt like we'd hit the jackpot; we felt like we would surely find the best of the best and exactly what we needed in his office.

My first appointment with the urogynecologist went well. He seemed confident that my issue was largely due to vaginismus (involuntary contraction of the vaginal muscles). He recommended the use of vaginal dilators at home to stretch out the muscles. So, I ordered a set of dilators online and committed to two months of daily use. I was to see him for a follow-up a couple of months later in mid-June.

Vaginal Dilators

Vaginal dilators are tube-shaped devices designed to stretch the vagina. Often made of medical-grade silicon, dilators come in various sizes. A small dilator might be the size of a tampon. A large one might be the size of an average penis. Dilators are used for a variety of conditions including, but not limited to, vestibulodynia, vaginismus, and during radiation treatment for gynecological cancers. Dilators may be obtained by prescription or purchased over-the-counter. A medical professional can teach women how to use dilators and tailor therapy to their personal situation[3].

International Society for Sexual Medicine

A BROKEN HEART

One week before that follow-up appointment and merely two days before our son's first birthday, our lives took another dramatic turn. Alan called from work late that Wednesday afternoon and said, "My chest and arm hurt. I think I'm having a heart attack." Against my warning, he drove himself home from work and I rushed him to the nearest urgent care. Instead of taking him seriously, they diagnosed him with heartburn and sent him out the door with an antacid.

Thankfully, we did not trust their diagnosis and proceeded to the emergency room of our go-to hospital where they rushed him through a battery of tests, the last of which was a heart catheterization. When the doctor called from the cath lab to tell me he found major arterial blockage and placed three stents in my 28-year-old husband's heart, I momentarily panicked. The previous 18 hours had been such a whirlwind. My sister-in-law sat in the hospital room with me; my husband's parents were out of state with their own medical crisis: Alan's mom was fighting breast cancer. About that time, a kind and knowledgeable nurse entered the room and patiently answered all of our questions. I quickly regained my composure and took a breath, just in time for my father-in-law to return my phone call.

Of all the trying things I had to do in my 26 years, that moment was by far the most difficult. How was I supposed to tell Alan's father that his son was in a hospital back home recovering from a heart attack? I couldn't compose myself enough to speak to him, so I handed the phone to my sister-in-law who, with God's strength, was able to save me and break the news to Alan's parents.

Needless to say, our entire family was more than thrilled to be home in our small town the next day–which happened to be our son's first birthday!

It sounds crazy, but as things settled we realized just how blessed we were. With the amount of blockage Alan had, he could have easily had a much more severe, damaging, or even fatal heart attack in a geographic location much further from a hospital.

In addition, Alan's heart attack combined with his mother's cancer diagnosis kickstarted my quest for truth in all areas of health and wellness.

BACK TO TREATMENT

Those major health events also put our sexual struggles into perspective. We needed to keep searching for an answer, but at the same time, we were thankful I did not have a life-threatening or debilitating illness.

My follow-up visit that next week with Dr. #4 was so-so. After using the dilators for two months, the doctor confirmed that the muscles surrounding my vaginal opening were significantly less tight. Unfortunately, as was the case after the intense pelvic floor rehabilitation in Florida, even though my pain minimized, it was still present. Intercourse continued to be uncomfortable; not unbearable, but not tolerable.

Treatment #4: Fail.

Dr. #4's next recommendation–still with no diagnosis, mind you–was a different type of pelvic floor PT. This time the PT treatment integrated biofeedback (a training tool to help patients learn to control muscle function[4]). I followed his recommendation with a local PT, but after two more months of treatment, there was no significant improvement.

Treatment #5: Fail.

I was just about ready for Dr. #4's next course of treatment–a steroid cream–when low and behold I became pregnant again. It really was mind-boggling that I could get pregnant so easily when we rarely had intercourse.

Sadly, the recurring pregnancies seemed to diminish the validity of my pain in the eyes of doctors. As I said before, the pregnancy phenomenon had to have something to do with my theory about ovulation. Whatever the case, we were thrilled to have another child even if pregnancy put the brakes on finding a pain solution.

Our precious, perfect daughter was born a few months later. Things rocked along crazy busy with an infant and a

Topical Steroids

In general, topical steroids are creams, ointments, or lotions which contain steroid medications and are most commonly used in the treatment of skin conditions to reduce skin inflammation and irritation. They come in different potencies and the greater the strength, the greater the risk of side-effects with continued use.[5] Though not indicated for most forms of vulvodynia or vestibulodynia (see Chapter 6), doctors with limited knowledge of the condition tend to prescribe topical steroids in an attempt to resolve a woman's symptoms.

toddler. We were extremely thankful for the health and happiness of our gifts from God.

When I'd had sufficient time to heal from my third C-section, Dr. #3 referred me to a local pain management doctor (Dr. #5) who specialized in treating women with pelvic pain. Of all the healthcare providers we had seen to that point, he was by far my favorite. His compassion was genuine and his desire to help was evident from the moment he stepped into the room. He radiated kindness.

Dr. #5's demeanor was the only reason I let him carry out his initial treatment recommendation: Steroid injections–*in my vagina*. Typically, I would have freaked out at the thought of needles being poked in that area, but after having an amniocentesis (giant needle in my belly to withdraw amniotic fluid) with our first child, the steroid treatment was bearable.

Unfortunately, the injections were unsuccessful. His next recommendation was topical lidocaine to numb the vestibule. No luck with that either. The final step was a pudendal nerve block. Basically, the doctor used ultrasound to guide a needle through my back to the pudendal nerve and administer anesthesia to numb the nerve.

Recalling and recording all these treatments on paper makes me realize I experienced a lot of less-than-fun treatments. In the end, the pain management doctor pulled many tricks out of his hat and some of those tricks lessened the

Steroid Injections

For women with certain forms of vestibulodynia, the use of injectible steroids in the vestibule provides pain relief. Some doctors prefer corticosteroids, while others prefer glucocorticoids. The goal is the same no matter the steroid injected - to reduce inflammation and thus relieve pain.

Pudendal Nerve Block

Pudendal nerve blocks are a minimally invasive, non-surgical treatment for chronic pain. These nerve blocks can help in the diagnosis of chronic pelvic pain conditions. In addition, pudendal nerve blocks can provide therapeutic relief by reducing pain signals originating from those nerves. When performed by pain management specialists, pudendal nerve blocks are performed with x-ray guidance to increase the accuracy and safety of the procedure.[6] Occasionally, gynecologists or sexual medicine physicians perform localized pudendal nerve blocks directly into the vestibular tissue for diagnostic purposes.

intensity of my pain; however, none of them provided complete relief.

Treatments #6, #7, and #8 – Fail, fail and fail.

As I stated before, my pain was neither chronic nor excruciating. Nevertheless, it was very real and very life-altering. All I could think with any sort of penetration was, "Get that out!" After five years, that physiological message began to have a significant negative impact on the emotional piece of our marriage.

FIRST TASTE OF PSYCHOTHERAPY

We knew the strain on our marriage was increasing and with a lack of physiological progress, we decided to search for help in the mental health world. It is unfortunate to note that after six years riddled with highly intense struggles, not one healthcare provider suggested we seek counseling. Thankfully, Alan and I were aware we needed help and both open to the potential benefits of psychotherapy.

Cognitive Behavioral Therapy

First, CBT is not the type of therapy in which you lie on a couch several times a week and dissect your dreams and your relationship with your mother. Instead, it is based on the idea that how you think about things directly affects how you feel and behave. It is a limited-time therapy, typically lasting for ten to twelve sessions, with each session highly structured and focused on a particular area. A major goal of CBT for therapists treating patients who are in pain is to change how the patient thinks about his or her pain in order to change how the pain feels. Studies find that CBT can be as effective as medication for a variety of mental health conditions, including mood, anxiety, personality, and substance abuse disorders. Studies also find it is quite effective for sexual pain. Keep in mind, however, that not all therapists deal with pain, and even fewer deal with both pain and sexuality[7].

When Sex Hurts

Much to our surprise, we quickly found a Christian marriage and family therapist who specialized in sex therapy, and decided to give the traditional Cognitive Behavioral Therapy a shot. While it was beneficial to be able to discuss such personal issues openly with a professional who truly understood the negative impact sexual problems could have on a relationship, the greatest benefit from our time with that therapist was a book he recommended we read as we searched for answers: *The Vulvodynia Survival Guide*.

DIAGNOSIS: VULVODYNIA

That first therapist's book recommendation led us to a self-prescribed diagnosis: *Vulvodynia*. Finally, a recognized condition. The descriptions and stories and treatments about which we read on those pages gave us the strength to con-

> **Vulvodynia**
>
> "Vulvodynia is a broad term used to describe any chronic pain in the vulvar area that lasts for at least three months. The term encompasses a variety of conditions with similar symptoms including Vestibulodynia/Vulvar Vestibulitis Syndrome."
>
> *The Vulvodynia Survival Guide*[8]

tinue searching; to keep hoping a little while longer. We still did not have all the answers, but we were so, so close. Or so we thought.

With our new-found knowledge and possible diagnosis, I returned to Dr. #3 after our daughter's first birthday to present my "case." She knew me well by that point. In the previous four years, between three high-risk pregnancies and trying to solve my pain issue, I was in her office at least monthly. So, when I mentioned that I had a self-diagnosis of Vulvodynia, she listened. I shared that we'd tried most of the treatments listed in *The Vulvodynia Survival Guide*, but not all. One option we had not yet tried was surgery. Much to my astonishment, she told me she had performed quite a few of those surgeries and believed it was a good option for me.

Looking back, I should have asked a few more questions before I agreed to surgery. However, there was (and still is) so little information available about this sort of condition for both patients and doctors, that I'm not sure what I would have asked.

A few weeks later, with complete faith and trust in Dr. #3's knowledge and abilities, I underwent what I thought was a vestibulectomy (more on that in Chapter 5). Recovery was quick and uneventful. I only needed a day or two to recover. We had a six-week hiatus before we could attempt intercourse, which would be the true test, of course. So, after six weeks, we gave it a go. Much to our dismay, it STILL hurt. How was it possible to still have pain? I kept thinking, "If cutting the tissue out didn't help, what more can we try?" From what I'd read, surgery was the final option; we were done. Talk about feeling hopeless–we were there.

Treatment #9: Fail.

HOPELESS

We had nowhere left to turn at that point. I kept searching for answers, but we began building a house two months after that surgery. And I literally mean building a house, with our own hands. so our time and minds were occupied. Between Alan working his day job and working on the house in the evenings, and raising a three-and-a-half and one-and-a-half-year-old, our life was craziness.

Despite all that, guess what happened in December? You guessed it–I became pregnant again. I have no idea how it happened. It goes back to my ovulation theory ... must have been just the right time. We were shocked, but it did not take long to become excited about our blessing.

Of course, pregnancy meant putting treatment on hold once again. Not that we had any options. In reality, life was so hectic between building a home, raising toddlers, and being pregnant and exhausted, there wasn't time to think about much else.

As if that fourth pregnancy wasn't stressful enough already, I developed a partial placenta previa, making me extra high-risk given our 30-minute drive to the nearest hospital. The high-risk obstetrician told me I would need to stay in the hospital from 32 weeks on since I lived so far away. She said that if the placenta tore and I began to bleed, I could bleed to death before I reached a hospital. I went into panic mode. Thankfully, Dr. #3 called me less than 30 minutes after my appointment with the high-risk OB and assured me I didn't need to check into the hospital; I would be okay at home. Even so, I remained on high alert the next two months and was equally relieved and elated when our second, healthy baby girl arrived via C-section at 38 weeks.

RAY OF HOPE

At that point in our lives, if things had been up to me, I would have given up. I was hopeless after the failed surgery; I was tired from life in general. My innate tendency when it came to emotionally-challenging events was to ignore them–to "move on." I told Alan that I did not have the mental or emotional strength to keep searching for solutions that didn't help and doctors who did not seem to care. Add to that, life with three kids under the age of four was a whirlwind of exhaustion. However, I remained willing to try any new treatments he found. I am grateful Alan kept looking, kept searching for someone to help us. His quiet strength and patience amazed me then and continues to amaze me now.

After a few months, his strength and searching paid off. He found another local therapist who specialized in sexual issues. While we both knew there was a very real physical problem, we recognized the psychological toll it continued to take on our relationship as well.

As usual, God provided help in His perfect timing. We met with a new therapist who provided the ray of hope we so desperately needed. She recommended something we had not considered in seven years–discovering ways to enhance our relationship until we could find a solution to the pain. It was one of those light-bulb moments. We had become so focused on the future, so focused on finding a solution, that we were not utilizing the strengths and abilities we had in the present. Small things like making time for each other, kissing, holding hands–all the little things that fall by the wayside while raising kids and living life. Not to mention living a life without intercourse. I hated to stop seeing her because she had so many great suggestions, but after a few months of listening and learning it was time for us to grow up and get to work for ourselves. So, we did, and our relationship grew much stronger as a result.

MY OWN ADVOCATE

As I mentioned in Chapter 2, I learned some invaluable lessons from childhood through early adulthood. Lessons that enabled me to achieve a variety of goals and earn the respect of employers and peers. For those lessons, I am eternally grateful. However, in contrast, as I became an adult, a wife, a mother, and faced the issue of unresolved sexual pain, I began to question one of those childhood teachings: that doctors have all the answers; that they are infallible. If they were so infallible, such experts, why did I still have unanswered questions? Why couldn't someone diagnose and treat me? Why, after eight years, was I still plagued with pain?

What I did not recognize at the time was that I had developed a new belief. I learned to become my own advocate. Only I knew the pains, feelings, and emotions running through my body. Alan and I both realized it was up to us and only us to keep looking, researching, and pressing on until we found someone who believed us and was willing to help. Coincidentally, as Americans in the new digital age, we were transitioning to a time when it was possible to find just about anything on the internet, and I was confident Alan and I had just as much ability as anyone else–doctor or layperson–to gather and decipher information.

So, we pressed on.

SECTION TWO:

to Educate

Be patient. Just like a puzzle, it takes time for all the pieces of your life to come together.
Unknown

5

To the West We Go

Disease in man is never exactly the same as disease in an experimental animal, for in man the disease at once affects and is affected by what we call the emotional life. Thus the physician who attempts to take care of the patient while he neglects this factor is as unscientific as the investigator who neglects to control all of the conditions that affect his or her experiment … One of the essential qualities of the clinician is interest in humanity, for the secret of care is in caring for the patient.

Francis Peabody, MD

Time stood still that September night as we scrolled through the pages of *When Sex Hurts: A Woman's Guide to Banishing Sexual Pain*. We sat in astonishment as, page by page, hope inched its way back into our hearts. When we got to the flowchart on pages 82-83 of the book, we knew it was a gift from God; an answer to our prayers.

Alan found *When Sex Hurts* earlier that day while combing the internet in desperation. After reading the first few pages, it was evident the book's authors–Dr. Andrew Goldstein, MD; Caroline Pukall, PhD; and Dr. Irwin Goldstein, MD–were the pioneers of sexual medicine and more specifically, as addressed in the book, dyspareunia (painful intercourse). How had we missed such a pertinent book in our years of searching? Simple: It was just published that year.

After a bit more digging around the internet we discovered Dr. Irwin Goldstein offered free courtesy calls to new patients–very impressive. So, the next morning I called his clinic, San Diego Sexual Medicine (SDSM), and set up a phone appointment.

It was tough to wait those nine days, but the wait was absolutely worth it. The 10 minutes I spent on the phone with the doctor were literally life-changing. His knowledge, kindness, and compassion were second to none as we discussed my symptoms, life, a potential diagnosis, tests, and a visit to SDSM. Nothing calms the anxiety of visiting a sexual medicine clinic quite like the excitement of visiting the Pacific Ocean on the same trip–at least for a land-locked girl like me.

Sexual Medicine

Sexual medicine attempts to improve sexual health through the prevention, diagnosis, treatment, and rehabilitation of conditions or diseases that involve sexual function.

Irwin Goldstein, MD, San Diego Sexual Medicine

SDSM ROUND #1

Because Alan was about to start a major project at work, we had to wait three months before we made our first trip to San Diego. That gave me time to complete the blood work Dr. Goldstein requested, gather medical records, and do more research to ensure it was a path we were willing to travel. Of course, I was kidding myself, Alan and I both agreed there was no doubt God was directing our steps West.

At this point, only Alan's mom, brother and sister-in-law knew we had a problem. I hadn't told a soul, but Alan told them. So, when it was time for that first trip to San Diego, we simply told everyone we were getting away for a short vacation. Which was somewhat true. It was the first trip we took alone since our children were born.

The moment we arrived in San Diego, I fell in love. It boasts perfect weather, a perfect ocean, perfect seafood, perfect produce grown year-round … I was even impressed with the city's roads and transportation. Maybe my instant connection to the city was based on the hopeful anticipation of a solution for my pain, but more likely it was the cool, dry air and soothing sound of the ocean waves. We had time that day to explore downtown, settle into our hotel on the bay, and find some great food in the Gaslamp Quarter.

The next day was the big day–our first visit with Dr. Goldstein (who is fondly referred to as Dr. G) and his incredible staff. Our wait in the lobby was short; Dr. G *himself* came to greet us and lead us to his office. He sat at his desk as Alan and I sat comfortably across from him. We discussed my history–when the pain began, attempted treatments, what made it better or worse, etc. Dr. G had dual computer monitors, including one that faced us, on which he showed illustrations of female anatomy as he explained potential causes of my pain. He truly wanted us to understand my body.

I was in awe at Dr. G's interest in our lives, conversational demeanor, and willingness to answer any question we wanted to ask. As we felt his genuine care and compassion not only for me, but also for Alan, the weight of the burden we had carried nearly silently for more than eight years began to lift.

As we had discussed on the phone, based on my history and the chart found on pages 82-83 of *When Sex Hurts*, my diagnosis was likely Congenital Neuroproliferative Vestibulodynia, but it was time to find out for sure. Alan and I were led to an exam room where I changed into a stylish paper gown.

Dr. G's nurse practitioner began the first portion of the physical exam–a vulvoscopy–by using a camera as a microscope to zoom in on the vulvar/vestibular tissue and look for abnormalities. The camera was connected to a television monitor on the wall, which enabled Dr. G, Alan, and I to see exactly what the NP could see. She also took still shots during the exam to save in my office file for future reference.

Congenital Neuroproliferative Vestibulodynia

Congenital Neuroproliferative Vestibulodynia is the result of an aberrant migration of neurons into the vestibule in greater than normal numbers. This results in an extremely high concentration of sensory nerve cells that are almost hyperactive in the way they relay tactile sensation. Much like other areas of the body, nerve hyperactivity causes nerve pain (neuropathy), often presenting as burning or stinging. By definition, women with primary NP-PVD have pain, and always have had pain, with insertion of any object–tampon, finger, penis, speculum–into the vagina, and approximately 60% of them will also have referred pain/discomfort in their umbilicus (belly button).

Contribution by Corey Babb, DO

The redness and inflammation of my vestibular glands were evident to even my untrained eyes. The vestibule's appearance combined with the extreme pain I felt when she performed the cotton swab test led them to confirm that I did, indeed, have a form of vestibulodynia.

Cotton Swab Test

The cotton swab test, or Q-tip test, is the current standard vulvodynia assessment for diagnosing provoked vestibulodynia. This test consists of using a cotton swab to palpate multiple vulvar and vestibular sites in a randomized fashion to control for sensitization while recording the woman's pain ratings upon palpation. The vestibule is organized into locations based on a clock face where the urethral meatus is at 12:00 and the 6:00 position is the posterior fourchette. A classic reading would be that the individual with a sexual pain history and consideration for vulvodynia would have, for example, a pain rating of 5/10 at the 1:00 position, while at the 9:00 position she may have a pain rating of 10/10. At the 5:00 position, she may have a pain rating of only 2/10. Traditionally, all clock regions 1:00, 3:00, 5:00, 6:00, 7:00, 9:00 and 11:00 are randomly tested and given pain ratings. There are many variations that health care providers use, as long as each provider uses a reproducible system to map out the regions of the vestibule and vulva along with the simultaneous documentation of the patient's pain rating.[1]

Andrew Goldstein, MD
Centers for Vulvovaginal Disorders

After the physical exam, I changed back into my clothes and we stepped down the hall to the office of Dr. Rose Hartzell, LMFT and AASECT Certified Sex Therapist. She had a kind, quiet demeanor–listening intently as we shared our eight-and-a-half-year journey. Toward the end of our time with her she made a single recommendation. That recommendation was to move our three children out of our bedroom (where they'd slept since we built our house) to give us more opportunity for intimacy. We readily complied with her recommendation when we returned home.

After we met with Dr. Hartzell, Dr. G escorted us a few doors down the hall to a pelvic floor physical therapist, Debbie Cohen, for her evaluation and treatment recommendations. Her sympathy for our situation and expertise in her field was as top-notch as everyone else in the office. We left our visit with a few suggestions for exercises I could begin at home.

After making our rounds, we landed back in Dr. G's office to discuss the day's events and develop a treatment plan. One treatment I had yet to try was hormone therapy. My calculated free testosterone level was low (see Chapter 6; serum testosterone and free testosterone are not the same), and because it was such a simple treatment with mild side effects, he wanted me to try hormone therapy to rule out hormonally-mediated vestibulodynia. I opted for a topical testosterone gel, as well as a cream I would directly apply to the vestibule daily.

Once we agreed on a game plan and exchanged goodbye hugs, we journeyed out to explore more of sunny San Diego and enjoy the rest of our last "us" day before returning home to our kiddos.

Out of the blue, after we were home a few days, Alan asked, "How do they do that?" To which I responded, "What are you talking about?" He answered, "How do they have everyone you need right there together?" He was referring to the office set-up at SDSM. Theset-up at SDSM blew my mind as well. The concept of having an assortment of providers in one location was simple, but rare. It served as proof of their understanding of the mind-body connection and the imperativeness of a holistic approach when addressing physiological concerns. When you add to that the love and care exuded by every member of the staff–to say we were blessed would be a vast understatement.

I began the prescribed topical testosterone therapy. Two months later I had blood drawn to evaluate the treatment's effectiveness. The good news was that my serum levels had improved. However, the real test was intercourse or provocation of the area, and unfortunately that was still painful.

Treatment #10: Fail.

Before we left San Diego the first time, Dr. G discussed the course of treatment we would take next if the hormone therapy failed to alleviate my pain. Alan and I would return to SDSM for a vestibular anesthesia test (basically numbing of the entire vestibule). In short, if my pain disappeared when my vestibule was numb, that would be a positive indicator that surgical removal of the vestibule–via complete vestibulectomy–should relieve my pain.

You're probably thinking, "Didn't you already have a surgery for this?" And that is correct. I thought I had a vestibulectomy three years prior. But, when Dr. G read through my operative notes from Dr. #3, she listed that surgery as a "skinny vulvectomy."

What exactly was a skinny vulvectomy? We had no idea. What we did know was that when Dr. G performed his first physical exam it was clear I still had a vestibule. The downside: I had an unnecessary surgery. The upside: surgery was still an option.

Since we knew I did not have hormonally-mediated vestibulodynia and we knew I did still have a vestibule, it was time to consider the next step, the VAT. While making another trip to San Diego was a bit tricky and quite expensive, deciding to move ahead with the VAT was simple. I mean, how many other times does a doctor give you a chance to "test" a surgical outcome before performing the surgery? I scheduled our next trip for two months later.

In the meantime, Dr. G sent me names, email addresses, and phone numbers of women who had walked that road before me. Just one more thing that made me appreciate Dr. G and SDSM: He continually desired and provided ways for me to be more informed than I even knew I should be. From connecting me with other patients, to explaining anatomy, emailing me for updates (yes, Dr. G emailed me and other patients directly), to inquiring to be sure Alan and I were on the same page when making decisions. There was nothing hidden and he did not put himself on a pedestal, instead he was transparent and focused on healing the patient.

SDSM ROUND #2

We decided to work our second trip to SDSM into a family vacation. Our son–five years old at the time–was fascinated with jets and ocean animals, so it was the perfect destination for him. In addition, it was an easy explanation for such a quick return to San Diego. We chose to leave our youngest child, who was one at the time, with my mother-in-law so we could travel easier and focus on our older two.

Our trip was perfect. We spent a couple of days exploring SeaWorld, LegoLand, and the San Diego Zoo before my appointment at SDSM. The day of that appointment I was a little nervous about my kids and what they might ask while we were there, but they were fantastic. They quietly watched a movie which allowed Alan to be with me during the VAT. Most of the time, those little moments/blessings in life have the greatest impact.

The NP and Dr. G both raved about a new, long-lasting numbing agent they were using with patients that would keep the treatment area numb for three days. Three days of numbness sounded great to me. I had no doubt that would give me plenty of time to decide whether surgery would be worth it.

Before she began the VAT, Dr. G's NP performed another cotton swab test to serve as the baseline of my vestibular pain pre-VAT. She then thoroughly explained the VAT procedure. I was surprisingly calm considering the fact that she was about to stick needles into my vagina–which makes me tense and squeamish all over again as I write these words. On the bright side, once she began, the numbing solution took effect and provided relief for the remainder of the procedure. While I don't want to relive the experience, it was bearable.

Following the injections, the NP performed another cotton swab test around each of the glands and had me rate my pain again. To my amazement, I didn't feel a thing. I did have some internal muscle tenderness, but I knew that was not uncommon for women with pelvic pain. Pelvic floor hypertension is quite often a secondary diagnosis for women with any type of vulvodynia. But, there was ZERO pain in the vestibular glands. The consensus was a positive VAT, indicating that a complete vestibulectomy would successfully eliminate my pain.

Anticipating three days' worth of numbness to do a little more experimenting with things like, well, intercourse, we decided to take our kids to the bay area to see fighter jets on an aircraft-carrier-turned-museum and on a boat ride through the harbor. We had a blast until the kids began to tire. We returned to our hotel and put a movie on for the kids, then went to another room in our suite to "experiment." I decided to try inserting a tampon first because I knew I would mentally anticipate pain with intercourse. Much to our dismay, that felt terribly painful. We were devastated; what an emotional let-down. Being the ever-optimistic, pillar-of-a-spouse he continually was, Alan suggested we replicate the cotton swab test. So we did, and discovered the pain in my vestibular glands had returned. Though completely unexpected, it was almost a relief to know it was the original pain and not something entirely different.

Because it was a Friday evening, I couldn't simply return to their office, so I emailed both the NP and Dr. G. Through email correspondence, we concluded that my body metabolized the numbing medication at an alarmingly quick rate, but we agreed the numbness in the office was enough to confirm a positive VAT test. So, while our balloon of excitement was deflated, we still knew where to go from there – a complete vestibulectomy.

As he did before the VAT, Dr. G provided contact information for numerous ladies with whom I could speak about my impending surgery. I emailed many of them and spoke by phone with a few of them. Although their experiences varied greatly, the consensus was that they were each happy with their decision to have surgery. Speaking with them sealed the deal–surgery it would be.

CARE OF THE PATIENT

At the beginning of this chapter I shared a statement by Dr. Francis Peabody from the 1927 March issue of the Journal of American Medicine that ended with "… for the secret of care is in caring for the patient." Dr. G knew that secret.

Complete Vestibulectomy

Vestibulectomy surgery is called complete right and left anterior and posterior vestibulectomy with vaginal advancement flap. Using this nomenclature, the complete surgery involves an excision of the portion of the vestibule that is several centimeters to the right and left above the urethral opening, called the urethral meatus. The complete surgery removes the entire lateral hymenal tissues to the lateral vestibular walls at Hart's line, and involves removal of the entire posterior fourchette from the posterior hymenal remnants down to the perineum. This wide excision is necessary to remove the high density of pain nerve fibers confined to the vestibular tissues that are not found in the vulvar or vaginal tissues. The high density of nerve fibers is derived from congenital neuronal hyperplasia as in primary provoked vestibulodynia or trauma/inflammation/genetic-induced neuronal hyperplasia as in secondary provoked vestibulodynia. The nerves are fortunately very near the skin surface so only a depth of 3 mm of vestibular skin needs to be excised. The usual surgical time is 60 minutes[2].

Sex in the 21st Century

At that point in our journey, my only real reservation about surgery was that it seemed like my final shot. What if it did not alleviate my pain? Would I just be out of luck and spend the rest of my life unable to have intercourse? In typical Dr. Goldstein fashion, when I shared my concern with him he came back with a quick, simple answer: "Then we will find something else that will work for you. We will not give up on you and will continue trying until we find a way for you to be pain-free." Wow. About the time I thought I could not be more impressed by the man, he one-upped himself. So many doctors are reactive. You make an appointment; they treat you; if that treatment does not help, you call to make another appointment; then they assume if you do not come back, their treatment recommendation was a success. There is typically no follow-up. Certainly no emails asking, "How are you doing?"

Dr. G is an exception. He thrives on and succeeds by knowing what works and what doesn't. To know that, he must communicate with his patients.

Hearing him say, "We will not give up on you," gave me the emotional relief and strength to prepare for surgery with hope and optimism. I had no doubt he would be there to help as long as I needed.

6

Provoked Vestibulodynia

I often say now I don't have any choice
whether or not I have Parkinson's,
but surrounding that non-choice is
a million other choices that I can make.
Michael J. Fox

Note: This chapter authored by Dr. Corey Babb.*

Provoked vestibulodynia (PVD) is the most common cause of sexual pain in the United States. It's estimated that up to 25 percent of women suffer from this condition[1], which is characterized by exquisite pain in the vulvar vestibule in response to physical stimulation. This stimulation doesn't have to be sexual–many women report their first episodes of PVD with gynecologic exams or tampon insertions. But when PVD occurs in conjunction with sexual activity, the results can be devastating.

In order to fully discuss PVD, a little background is needed. First, a definition. If you break the word vestibulodynia apart, *-vestibulo-* relates to the vulvar vestibule, the anatomic area between Hart's Line and the Hymenal ring, and -*dynia*-, which simply means "pain." The term 'provoked vestibulodynia' is actually the amalgamation of a number of disorders previously labeled vulvovestibulitis syndrome (VVS), vulvodynia, or just plain ol' vestibulitis. Nowadays, however, we use the term PVD to include any type of provoked pain in the vulvar vestibule, regardless of etiology.

Now that we've defined PVD, we can talk about different causes of the disease. PVD is categorized based on its root pathology, which may be inflammatory, hormonal, infectious, or neuroproliferative in origin. Unfortunately, this variety of potential causes can make the disorder difficult to treat - a truth many frustrated patients have experienced firsthand. In order to better understand the origins of the disorder, let's look at each cause individually.

INFLAMMATORY PVD

Inflammatory PVD is due to a localized inflammatory response in the vulvar vestibule. This may be due to inflammatory skin conditions such as Lichen Sclerosis or Psoriasis, or allergic responses to detergents, clothes, or bath products. In some cases, Inflammatory PVD resolves if the root cause is removed. This may be a simple fix, as in the case of allergic responses. However, skin conditions, such as Lichen Sclerosis, are much more difficult to treat, often requiring months or even years of therapy.

One especially frustrating, albeit significantly rare, type of inflammatory PVD, is a condition called Desquamative Inflammatory Vaginitis (DIV). As a whole, DIV is poorly understood, with research into the condition being sparse at best. What we do know, however, is that DIV occurs as a response to some external stimuli, possibly a bacterial or fungal invasion, and causes an impressive "sloughing" of the vestibular and vaginal epithelium (outer most tissue layer).

Women suffering from DIV complain of excessive vaginal discharge, which often "sticks to underwear like glue." This discharge is not necessarily smelly or irritating on its own but causes vaginal, vestibular, and vulvar tissue to become red and inflamed due to constant moisture. Once a diagnosis is made, treatment usually involves the use of high-potency steroids in the form of creams, ointments, or injections. In the case of DIV, antibiotics may be especially useful as well.

HORMONAL PVD

Hormonal PVD occurs as a response to an imbalance of hormones within the cells of the vestibule. Surprisingly, the hormone usually responsible for Hormonal PVD is testosterone. How does this happen? Embryologically speaking, the cells that form the vaginal vestibule in women are homologous to the cells that form the prostate in men. These cells are rich in androgen receptors, and depend on testosterone to grow and properly function. This is why certain chemotherapies for prostate cancers deprive the prostate of its ability to take up and use testosterone.

Obviously, women don't have to worry about prostate cancer, but androgen receptors in the vestibule can experience changes in a low-testosterone state, namely inflammation, involution, and alterations in cellular biology. Clinically speaking, this hormonal deprivation causes significant redness and can lead to intense burning, itching, or searing pain with stimulation. Now, most women are not taking chemotherapy agents, especially ones targeting testosterone receptors. What may surprise you, however, is that anti-testosterone medications, also known as anti-androgens, are actually very common the world of gynecology. So common in fact that 16% of reproductive women take these medications daily[2]. Care to guess what medication type it is? If you guessed oral contraceptive pills (birth control pills), you're right Birth control pills increase the level of a hormone called Sex Hormone Binding Globulin (SHBG), whose main job is to pick up circulating "free" or "unbound" hormones, and prevents it from being used. In this case, high SHBG leads to low free testosterone. Low free testosterone leads to a hormonally deficient state in the vestibule, which is what we call Hormonal PVD. How do you fix this? First of all, stop taking the birth control pill. Secondly, replace testosterone. After about six weeks of testosterone therapy, most women with hormonal PVD secondary to birth control pill usage will note significant improvement in their symptoms.

But what if you're not using birth control pills? Many medications (Spironolactone, Leuprolide, flutamide, to name a few), physiologic states (menopause), and even surgeries such as an oophorectomy (removal of the ovaries) can cause a decrease in your testosterone. Luckily, treatment is more or less the same. Stop the offending agent if possible, and replace the deficient testosterone. Obviously certain cases–menopause, surgery–cannot be reversed, but supplementing testosterone should still yield a noticeable improvement in vestibular symptoms.

INFECTIOUS PVD

Infectious PVD is most commonly associated with certain types of sexually transmitted infections (STI's). Ulcerative STI's, such as herpes simplex virus (HSV), cause a localized breakdown in the skin layer and lead to painful lesions that sometimes ooze clear fluid. In the case of HSV, this fluid contains the viral particles that transmit the disease, so special care should be taken when patients with active lesions engage in sexual activity. Other infectious organisms include Staphylococcus aureus, Streptococcus species, and many types of yeast. As a general rule, diagnosis of infectious PVD is based on clinical findings and positive cultures of the infectious agent. Treatment should be focused on the type of infection and can include antibiotic, anti-fungal, or antiviral medication.

NEUROPROLIFERATIVE PVD

Neuroproliferative PVD is perhaps the most complex type of PVD, in both diagnosis and treatment. Many women who suffer from Neuroproliferative PVD (NPPVD) see multiple specialists before they are ever diagnosed correctly, and once the diagnosis is made, treatments are often trial-and-error in nature. To better understand NPPVD it is important to differentiate between primary and secondary subtypes. Unfortunately, this distinction is rarely made, and as such, many women are treated inappropriately, often undergoing unnecessary surgical intervention.

PRIMARY NEUROPROLIFERATIVE PVD

Primary (sometimes called congenital) neuroproliferative PVD is the result of an aberrant migration of neurons into the vestibule in greater than normal numbers. This results in an extremely high concentration of sensory nerve cells that are almost hyperactive in the way they relay tactile sensation. Nerve hyperactivity causes a certain type of pain (neuropathy), which often presents as burning, stinging, or, as one patient put it, "The sensation of shards of broken glass rubbing in my vagina." Women with primary NPPVD have pain, and always have had pain, with insertion of any object - tampon, finger, penis, speculum – into the vagina, and approximately 60 percent of them will also have referred pain/discomfort in their umbilicus (belly button). Treatment for primary NPPVD is focused on decreasing nerve activity in the vestibule. Medications such as gabapentin, amitriptyline, and duloxetine are first-line oral treatments for this condition, and in some women, are extremely helpful. Other women require injectable steroids or topical anesthetic agents, while some patients find that compounded topical versions of anti-inflammatory drugs - cromolyn and diclofenac, to name a few - are useful in treating their pain. If medical therapy does not work, women with primary NPPVD may benefit from surgical management in the form of a procedure called a vestibulectomy.

Now, let me be very clear. Primary NPPVD is the only form of PVD that benefits from surgical intervention. If your provider is recommending a vestibulectomy for any other type of PVD, please get a second opinion, preferably from someone who has experience in treating this condition. If, however, you are a candidate for a vestibulectomy, it is important to make sure that your surgeon has experience performing the procedure, with a good knowledge of appropriate aftercare following surgery. There's nothing worse than going through a procedure, only to end up no better off than you were before.

SECONDARY NEUROPROLIFERATIVE PVD

Secondary neuroproliferative provoked vestibulodynia is similar to primary NPPVD in terms of symptoms but differs in presentation history. Women with secondary NPPVD can recall a time when they were pain-free, and can often pinpoint an event or occurrence when they started having vestibular pain. Typically, vulvovaginal trauma in the form of infection, or childbirth is the culprit. In terms of treatment, localized steroid injection tends to work better with secondary NPPVD, but as always, results vary from patient to patient. As stated above, vestibulectomy is NOT indicated for secondary NPPVD.

HELP IS AVAILABLE

Regardless of the type of provoked vestibulodynia you have, I hope that this information is helpful to you. The unfortunate truth is that a great number of women's health providers not only commonly misdiagnose this disease but have little understanding of treatment options. The National Vulvodynia Association can be a wonderful resource for women who feel alone in their struggles with sexual and pelvic pain, and the International Society for the Study of Women's Sexual Health (ISSWSH) provides a list of providers worldwide who are knowledgeable in the diagnosis and treatment of vestibulodynia. A list of additional resources can be found in the back of this book – I encourage you to check them out if you still have questions.

In closing, while provoked vestibulodynia is a disorder that can affect not only your personal life but also the quality of intimate relationships you may have, it is not without treatment. Be persistent in seeking quality care, and if something sounds fishy, get a second opinion. You are always your best health advocate.

*Author: **Corey R. Babb**, D.O., FACOOG, IF, NCMP
Clinical Assistant Professor of Obstetrics and Gynecology
Director of Clinical Operations
Department of Obstetrics and Gynecology
Oklahoma State University College of Osteopathic Medicine

For a thorough **glossary** of sexual-medicine-related terms refer to the book *When Sex Isn't Good* by Sue Goldstein and Lillian Arleque.

For applicable **illustrations** of the female anatomy mentioned throughout this book see *When Sex Hurts* by Andrew Goldstein, M.D.; Irwin Goldstein, M.D.; and Caroline Pukall, Ph.D.

7.

My Vestibulectomy

Exceptional patients refuse to be victims.
They educate themselves and become
specialists in their own care. They question
the doctor because they want to understand
their treatment and participate in it.
They demand dignity, personhood, and control,
no matter what the course of the disease.
Bernie S. Siegel, MD

During the six months leading up to surgery, I spoke with women who had been through the surgery about their recoveries, conversed with Dr. G multiple times by phone and email, and read quite a few post-op stories written by his patients on an internet forum. I was grateful so many others would share their time and energy speaking with me and documenting their journeys so that those of us on similar paths would know what to expect.

Due to the abundance of information literally at my fingertips, I had very few questions for Dr. G during our four phone consultations before the surgery. I usually asked him to share what he believed to be most vital. The single concern I did have was the estimated six-week recovery. That seemed hard to imagine. In the previous six years I'd experienced and recovered from four C-sections. Those were major surgeries. I barely spent six weeks recovering from the four combined. And three of those times I went home with infants for whom to care. Six weeks of downtime seemed unfathomable. That amount of recovery time would require help from family and friends. Now don't get me wrong, there were lots of people who would have jumped to my aid. The problem was that I didn't want help; I hadn't even mentioned the surgery. I was a strong, independent woman who took pride in being in control. If I was going to have help, especially after a medical procedure, I only wanted my husband as my caregiver. I knew he would take care of me well. Realistically, though, he could not leave his job for more than one week.

Not only did I not want to need help, I honestly could not envision lying around for a month and a half. I could barely sit through an entire movie without getting up to do something or letting my mind wander down 100 different paths. In addition, our kids were 2, 4, and 6 at the time so they needed me. I simply could not wrap my mind around how I could manage a recovery of that length.

Back to my previous mention of reading post-op stories written by former patients … while most of the stories were highly beneficial, a few began to freak me out. I was well aware that one's mind could play a vital role in recovery. I understood Dr. G wanted me to be prepared heading into surgery. However, one day while reading a story from someone who said she didn't leave her house for 14 weeks following surgery I thought I was going to have a nervous breakdown. At that moment I chose to stop reading others' stories and start writing my own. I vowed to make my recovery as quick and successful as possible.

CHARTING MY COURSE

One year prior I'd joined a company that promoted whole-body wellness through lifestyle changes and food-based supplements. Utilizing the vast amount of knowledge about the human body and nutrition I'd worked so hard to gain through the years, I developed a plan regarding post-op foods and supplements to aid in my recovery (See Appendix A). After creating my game-plan, I made an appointment with my functional medicine physician, Dr. Chad Edwards. I shared the details of my surgery along with my recovery plan. He recommended I include three additional supplements, as well as IV nutritional therapy both pre-op and post-op. Once I had a thorough nutritional plan in place my anxiety disappeared.

Functional Medicine

The focus in functional medicine (FM) is on understanding the origins, prevention, and treatment of complex, chronic disease. FM is comprehensive and integrative, considering how the entire body functions as a single organism. Disruption of any single component always affects something else. These changes cannot happen in isolation. Functional medicine considers the individual genetic makeup along with internal (mind, body, and spirit) & external (physical and social environment) factors that affect total body function. FM physicians understand that health is much more than the absence of disease. They incorporate western medical practice with alternative or integrative medicine. A primary focus is on prevention through the "healthy trinity" (exercise, nutrition, and the 3R's). FM physicians use the latest laboratory and diagnostic testing to identify underlying disruptions and incorporate prescription medications, supplements, herbal medicines, nutrition, detoxification, stress-management, and sleep optimization.

Contribution by Chad Edwards, D.O.
Revolution Health & Wellness

IV Nutritional Therapy

Optimal health requires sufficient nutrition. Unfortunately, we live in a time when nutritional deficiencies are common. Intravenous (IV) nutritional therapy can provide high doses of nutrients in a safe, beneficial, simple, and effective method. Advantages of IV nutritional therapy include immune support, higher blood levels, and a rapid effect. While the therapy can be tailored to address specific medial conditions, many patients benefit from what is known as a Myer's Cocktail. IV nutritional therapy is often recommended pre- and post-surgery; during recovery from athletic training events and/or competitions; and to help with allergies, drug withdrawal, depression, adrenal fatigue, and more.

Contribution by Chad Edwards, D.O.
Revolution Health & Wellness

However, the anxious feelings returned when I shared my plan with Dr. G during our final phone appointment before surgery. He was less than thrilled about it, especially the IV portion. My bubble of excitement burst. After I replayed our conversation in my mind for a couple of days, I humbly realized he was simply doing what he did best–striving to protect his patient. He had no way of knowing my nutrition experience or that Dr. Edwards was a sound physician and not a fly-by-night quack doctor. I composed an email explaining the reasoning behind my choices and that I would be sure they would not contribute to increased bleeding or cause other complications. In the end, he said he would support my decisions. Once again, my anxiety diminished, and I spent the remaining two days cleaning house and preparing for post-op simplicity.

SDSM ROUND #3

Time flew between trips number two and three. It was hard to believe it was already time to return to San Diego. The city stole my heart during our first trip, so I was thrilled to return, even for major surgery. Likewise, our kids were always excited to spend a couple of days with their grandma, so they were happy as clams when Alan and I left them to catch our evening flight West.

PRE-OP

After a short night, a scrumptious ocean-side breakfast, and a little sand between our toes, it was time for my pre-op appointment at Alvarado Hospital. Curious to know just how much I trusted Dr. G? Until that moment, I had not even considered researching the hospital. I was shocked that it was so small, but confident Dr. G demanded a superb operating room.

After the hospital pre-op, we made the short trip across the street to SDSM. Our first appointment there was with Dr. Hartzell, the therapist. We always seemed to leave her a bit speechless during our visits. When we left her office Alan said, "She doesn't know what to think about us." That was a very real possibility. I wasn't certain if her quietness meant she thought we didn't need much help or that we needed much more help than she could address in an hour. She did attempt to warn me that I might be expecting too quick a recovery. I admitted that it was possible I was being unrealistic, but I had always preferred to live life with a shoot-for-the-moon attitude.

When we finished with Dr. Hartzell, the NP performed one last vulvoscopy and cotton swab test to verify that I did, in fact, have pain in the vestibular glands. There was no doubt during that test that I still had pain. Once that was confirmed, we joined Dr. G in his office where he shared surgery photos and spent time explaining exactly what he would do during the next day's procedure. He took care to answer every question we had. Not once did we feel rushed, even though it was well after 5 p.m. when we left the clinic.

Alan and I were past ready for supper by that point. We chose a restaurant along the bay and enjoyed a fantastic dinner before we found a pharmacy to fill my prescriptions and shopped for comfortable pants for me to wear the next few weeks.

SURGERY DAY

Day 1 - It sounds crazy to say, but I was excited for surgery. I was completely confident it was the answer to lots of prayers and would be the key to ending painful intercourse. Plus, I've always liked a challenge, so I was ready to get past the surgery and have a quick recovery.

As is typical for any planned surgery, we checked in with the nurses in the pre-op office. Then Alan went to the waiting room while I changed, they took my vitals, and placed an IV. I was thankful they let Alan join me again at that point–I felt much better with him beside me. Dr. G came to check on us, as did a few of the OR staff. Finally, I met the anesthesiologist. I felt surprisingly calm at that point–probably from the medications. Dr. G was so anxious to begin that he helped wheel my bed into the OR. Once they got me onto the surgical table and administered the anesthesia, I was out.

POST-OP

The next thing I knew, I was coming-to in the post-anesthesia care unit. I always disliked the feeling of waking up from anesthesia, but I had a great nurse and I was in zero pain so waking that time wasn't terrible. In no time she had me up, getting dressed, and walking to the restroom. We did not need to be at the airport for two more hours, so Alan wheeled me downstairs and drove me over to SDSM where the office girls gave me water and helped me get comfy in one of their rooms. Shortly after settling in, I began feeling pain. Remember the numbing solution from the VAT that was designed to last three days but only hung with me about three hours? That was not a fluke. The three-hour mark seemed to be its limit this time as well. So, I took the first dose of my prescription pain medicine and the pain stabilized.

By that point it was time to head to the airport for our flight home. We said our goodbyes to the SDSM staff, got our hugs from Dr. G and his wife, Sue, then with my donut pillow and pain meds in tow, Alan wheeled me to the car where I stretched out in the back seat for the 15-minute ride. We returned the rental car, took the shuttle to the airport entrance, and quickly located a wheelchair. It was time to be on my A-game. I was certain if the airlines knew I was only four hours post-op they would not let me on a plane. I remember thinking before surgery that I would just be tough and walk. When the time came, I changed my tune and eagerly crawled in the wheelchair with my pillow and a smile. Navigating through security was a breeze. An attendant wheeled me to the front of the line and in less than five minutes we were headed to our gate.

Waiting to board our flight provided an opportune time to eat. I was not at all hungry, but since I'd already taken one pain pill, and Dr. G recommended I take another along with a sleeping pill before boarding the flight, I thought it wise to eat. By eat, I mean drink my favorite combination of orange juice/powdered greens/chia seeds and snack on a few pretzels. Make note of this, because it will come back up later in the story. I was quite the alternative-health nut and treated most problems with food, supplements, or oils. I rarely took mainstream medication. For this scenario, though, legitimate pain relief and sleeping sounded great.

Since I was in a wheelchair, we boarded the plane first. I was able make myself somewhat comfortable in a window seat with my life-saving pillow, fresh ice pack, and cozy blanket. I was ready for take-off. It was Oklahoma or bust.

The first flight was great until about halfway through, when all of a sudden I felt extremely heated, severely nauseous, my head began to spin, and I knew I was about to faint. All I could think was, "I've got to get out of here, I've got to get off this plane!!"

Remember me saying to make note of what I ate because it would come back up later? Well, it did, literally. Thankfully Alan grabbed a plastic bag in which I could lose my pretzels. Almost instantly my symptoms dissolved, and I survived the rest of that first flight without incident. When we switched planes in Denver, we called Alan's cousin, a pharmacist, to ask if I could take motion sickness medication on top of everything else I'd had that day. He said it would not cause problems, so I took a dose with a bit of ginger ale and slept most of the second flight.

HOME AT LAST

It was surreal to be in our car, headed home, four entire states away from where we started, just a little more than 12 hours after my surgery began. Per doctor's orders, as soon as we arrived home I headed upstairs for a warm, soothing bath. Finally, nurse Alan helped me into fresh clothes, unpacked my pain medicine, and helped me get situated in bed with pillows propping my legs just right and an ice pack on my incision.

Dr. G called Alan three times throughout the afternoon and evening to check on me. Once we settled in at home, Alan let him know I was still doing well.

That first night was uneventful–which was great since we'd had such a long day. Because I was so full of fluids from surgery, I did wake up two or three times with a full bladder. Not only was getting in and out of bed quite a feat, but also, the moment urine poured over that fresh wound it burned like fire.

Thankfully, I remembered a trick from my C-section days and found a perineal irrigation bottle I could fill with warm water, which I then used to rinse every time I needed to urinate. The warm water helped make it easier to go in the first place, and washed the acidity away from the incision.

RECOVERY

Day 2 - I woke up ready to see my kids. My pain level was low, especially after more pain meds and a bath. We actually made the 45-minute drive back to Tulsa that morning for my second IV treatment. Shortly after Dr. Edwards' nurse started my IV and helped me get comfortable, my pain began to escalate. In true perfect timing, Dr. G called my cell phone to check on me. He instructed me to take the pain medication more frequently than I had been. Even though that could increase constipation, pain management was top priority. Pain is such a hopeless feeling, even when sitting in the middle of a doctor's office. Thankfully my pain deescalated quickly, and by the time we left I felt much better.

Here's a funny "drugged" story: We stopped at a local bakery for chicken noodle soup. While Alan was inside getting our food, I called one of my best friends and told her about my surgery. There's nothing quite like narcotics to make you spill your secrets. I even told a few more people while I was drugged-up those first few days.

When we got home, I took another bath before an additional round of pain meds, ice, and a nap. When I woke up, our kiddos were all back home. My little sweeties were so gentle and loving with me. The rest of the day and night consisted of pain meds, warm baths (did I mention how amazing baths felt?), frequent icing, and talking with Dr. G. My pain level averaged a 3 out of 10–not bad, in my opinion.

Day 3 – As expected, the pain was a bit stronger the third day, but it was nothing the pain meds, ice, baths, and rest couldn't control. Dr. G called first thing that Saturday morning. His selflessness was incredible. How many other doctors spend their Saturday mornings calling patients? I established my food and supplement routine throughout the day (see Appendix A) and found a new yummy snack: Homemade applesauce mixed with pecan butter and Mila (chia seeds). It tasted like a pecan pie. By late afternoon, since I had not had a bowel movement in two days, Dr. G strongly encouraged I use an enema to get things moving. Constipation could lead to more pain, which I certainly wanted to avoid. It did the trick. A couple of times that day my pain jumped to a 7 or 8, but that was no match for warm water and ice.

Day 4 - Alan took our kids to church, so I had the house (or should I say bed) to myself for a while. The quiet was soothing, but I became lonely before they returned. My routine was the typical bed, bath, ice, pain meds, supplements, and a little food (smoothies, juices). My pain measured a consistent 2 or 3 throughout the day. For me, the worst side effect of the narcotics was a constant headache, so I began a successful transition from the prescription pain medication to over-the-counter acetaminophen and ibuprofen.

Day 5 - Same routine as Day 4. I spent more of the day out of my bed and on the couch which made it easier to interact with my kids. As you can tell, my recovery those first few days was pleasantly uneventful. Alan was an exceptional nurse. I would have enjoyed a little more time with him, but he had to balance hanging out with me versus letting me rest by keeping our kids quiet or outside.

Day 6 – For some reason I had a terrible time getting to sleep the night of Day 5. Shortly after I finally fell sleep, I woke up to extreme itching at my incision site. I dozed for a couple of hours before eventually getting in the bath at 5 a.m. After a 45-minute soak, I iced the area and took a sleeping pill (the first I had taken since boarding our flight home). Once the sleeping pill kicked in, I was able to sleep most of the day. By afternoon I was ready to venture out of the house, so I made the 30-minute trip with Alan to pick our girls up from school. I was happy to be out of the house but by the time we got back home I was exhausted. I also called Dr. G's NP in search of a solution for the unbearable itching. She ordered a prescription strength antihistamine from a local pharmacy. That medication served as a lifesaver during the remainder of my recovery.

Day 7 – Alan returned to work, so my mom took care of us for the day. Well, took care of our girls anyway. I was self-sufficient by that point. I bathed, iced, supplemented, and tried to find the sleep that kept eluding me. I eventually resorted to another sleeping pill, but it had surprisingly little effect.

Week 2 – One week down. Because we were so far from San Diego and follow-up appointments were unrealistic, the next best option was pictures. So, every couple of days Alan would photograph the surgery site and email the photos to Dr. G. Talk about double-, triple- and quadruple-checking the email recipient line–we did not want those photos sent to the wrong person. What a blessing, though, to live in a day and age when email, texting, and phone calls are the norm. It drastically narrowed our geographical divide.

To celebrate the one-week mark, we journeyed out for dinner at a nearby restaurant. Unfortunately, I continued to have trouble sleeping the next week or so. I started doing more housework, laundry, and cooking. I may have pushed a little too hard, because my pain increased some, but moving around was worth it.

By Sunday I was ready to join my church family for worship. Walking and sitting in manners that concealed my pain (because the majority of them had no idea I'd had surgery) required a bit of creativity.

My only real complaint at that point was the "brain fog" from anesthesia and medication. I was only 11 days post-op, but I had the bright idea later that afternoon to make a 40-mile drive to meet some friends who were anxious to hear about my nutrition business. Probably not my wisest decision ever, but it all worked out well. I was certainly ready to rest when I made it back home.

Before surgery I was nervous about the timing, but looking back it was perfect. Not only was I to avoid vaginal penetration of any kind for at least three months, Dr. G also strongly advised against sexual arousal *of any kind* to ensure the vestibular glands did not reform and create post-op complications. Alan began a major project at work that week which meant 14-hour work days, seven days a week. My recovery was not a cake walk for Alan, so being extra busy at work–leaving us little time together–was a good thing in disguise.

By the end of the second week I resumed grocery shopping and transporting my kiddos to and from school. Those activities were exhausting, but doable. While I would not categorize those first two weeks of recovery as fun, I was blessed considering I was recovering from a surgery that made walking, sitting, standing, and even lying down difficult and painful.

Week 3 – I felt extra fatigued and slightly congested toward the middle of the third week, so I went for another round of IV vitamin therapy. That was a great decision as it seemed to fast-track my healing from that point forward. One of my best friends made a trip to visit and clean house for me (she is wonderful like that)–and yet another case of perfect timing. The next night my sister and her family, along with some other good friends, came to our house for supper. We had a great time, but I was sure ready for my bath and bed that night.

BACK TO NORMAL

Week 4 – Then, just like that, the day arrived. Only 23 days post-op and I felt "normal." I had zero pain when sitting or walking. I continued ibuprofen to prevent pain, but the only prescription I consumed was the antihistamine to control itching as the tissue healed. I resumed my normal activities without trouble: Cleaning house, caring for kids, mountains of laundry, a hair appointment, lunch with a friend, etc. I worked hard to stay on top of things nutritionally, and I could tell my body was using less energy to recover and more energy for daily activities.

It felt great to knock that ball out of the park; to cut the projected six-week healing time nearly in half. Dr. G was consistently surprised at the rate of healing he observed through my photos.

At that point, the only lingering reminders of surgery were a few stitches and brain fog. Thankfully, the latter was no match for a combination of gentle detoxing/cleansing products and an adrenal-supporting energy drink.

Week 5 – For months I had planned to attend a company event in Dallas (a four-hour drive). I never had a doubt that I would be able to attend; nonetheless, I was still thrilled when the time came and I really did feel good enough for the trip. The two trickiest parts of the whole weekend were deciding what to wear (I still preferred soft, comfortable pants to jeans) and managing the long walk back and forth from the Omni Hotel to the convention center. Coincidentally, Dr. G happened to call that weekend and was nearly speechless when I explained where I was.

Even though my healing continued ahead of schedule, Dr. G suggested I wait until the three-month mark to begin the next phase of therapy: Pelvic floor rehab. However, he did clear me to begin external PT when I reached eight weeks post-op. At that time, there were four pelvic floor PTs practicing in Tulsa–unheard of in that size of city. What a blessing it was to have choices. I spoke with each of them, considered their office locations, chose the one I felt would be the best fit for me, and scheduled my first appointment.

PHYSICAL THERAPY

Although I knew what to expect from my previous pelvic floor PT experiences, I was nervous about the appointment. My nervesousness diminished quickly once I met my new PT, Becky. The first visit was simply an evaluation to determine the strengths and weaknesses throughout my musculoskeletal structure. She keyed in on my chronic back pain and sent me home with a list of exercises to increase hip strength and stabilization.

I continued weekly PT appointments for the next month. During that time, Becky and I worked to release tightness in my hips, realign my hips and spine, strengthen my core, and relieve any tension that could potentially contribute to pelvic floor dysfunction.

I had two more follow-up phone appointments with Dr. G that month, and I sent a few more photos to document my healing. There were times I literally sat in awe of the intricacy and complexity of the human body and its ability to heal. Truly the handiwork of a mighty Creator.

As we neared the three-month mark, I was long overdue for a good dose of "stress relief." Intercourse was still off limits, but we had plenty of experience reaching orgasm without intercourse, so we gave it a shot. It felt incredible, temporarily. A few seconds after I climaxed I felt a very sharp, clenching pain. Talk about an emotional roller coaster. I was at a very high, high and very low, low all within about five seconds–and so was Alan.

It took a couple of hours for the pain to subside. As painful, disappointing, and frustrating as that was, we had peace knowing Dr. G would have an answer or work to find one. When I spoke to him two days later, he knew just what to say. He was certain the pain was caused by my pelvic floor muscles going into spasm after they tightened during orgasm, and suggested we try again when I could focus on relaxing my pelvic floor muscles through breathing. A couple of nights later we followed his suggestion, and it worked. To say we were relieved would be an understatement.

By the end of the third month post-op, I was ready for the next step of recovery: Internal PT. Much to my surprise, the scar at my surgical site was not at all painful. Some of the deeper muscles were quite tight, but they released well. Though I was sore a day or two following that appointment, I was excited to start that leg of the journey as it meant we were one step closer to the finish line.

8

The Storm After the Calm

Count it all joy, my brothers, when you meet trials of various kinds, for you know that the testing of your faith produces steadfastness. And let steadfastness have its full effect, that you may be perfect and complete, lacking in nothing.
James 1:2-4

Alan wanted me to title this chapter *The Day My Vagina Swallowed a Purple Softball*. As you read about what happened next, keep in mind that we learned an important lesson we thought we already knew: Be extremely picky when choosing a doctor.

Throughout the fourth month post-op I continued to improve in physical therapy treatment; progressing easily to the third largest of four dilators. Between manual trigger-point release at home and the therapy Becky performed during appointments, my muscles were no longer going into spasm and seemed to stabilize and strengthen as they should.

We had yet to attempt intercourse. We could have, but I wanted to give myself the best possible chance to have zero pain. It was at that point in our journey that I began to see an "end" to our struggles with sexual pain for the first time in, well, ever.

That was short-lived, though, because the next month I began to have a new pain following orgasm. We were experts in emailing photos to Dr. G, so I immediately had Alan snap a photo of the painful area and sent it to him. He suspected Bartholin's cysts, which are not uncommon after a vestibulectomy, but only require treatment about 5 percent of the time[1]. Mysteriously, the left cyst was larger than the right cyst, but because it was deeper beneath the surface of my skin it was not painful. The cyst on my right side, though, looked like a blister and remained painful for at least 24 hours following orgasm. It was also especially painful when I walked.

Without hesitation, I made a phone appointment with Dr. G. He told me the larger, deeper cyst did not need treatment unless it began to cause pain. As for the smaller, painful cyst, he would prefer I make the trek to San Diego for treatment, but understood that the simple procedure needed to "unroof" the cyst might not warrant the time and expense necessary to make that trip. In his words, "Anyone should be able to take care of that one."

Bartholin's Cyst

The Bartholin's glands are located on each side of the vaginal opening. These glands secrete fluid that helps lubricate the vagina. Sometimes the openings of these glands become obstructed, causing fluid to back up into the gland. The result is relatively painless swelling called a Bartholin's cyst. Treatment of a Bartholin's cyst depends on the size of the cyst, how painful the cyst is, and whether the cyst is infected.[2]

IF I KNEW THEN WHAT I KNOW NOW

The ball was in my court, so to save a couple thousand dollars I chose to pursue treatment locally. After lots of research (and not nearly enough prayer) I chose Dr. #7. Alan accompanied me to my first appointment with him to help me decide if he was the right choice. Dr. #7 had a great bedside manner. I shared my notes, history, and current problem. He was curious about how we found Dr. G and seemed genuinely intrigued by our journey.

During the physical examination he said he wasn't sure what was causing my new pain, but that it couldn't be a Bartholin's cyst. He did not observe anything that could be causing the pain and eventually told me, "You may not ever be pain-free." Talk about taking the wind out of your sails ... I mustered the strength to ask a few questions, which he answered. Before we left that appointment, the doctor encouraged me to share his lack of findings with Dr. G.

I should have trusted my instincts to run far, far away from his office and never look back. Unfortunately, my faith in humanity coupled with my desperate need for pain relief, led me to request (per Dr. G's recommendation) an ultrasound of the areas where we believed the cysts were located. Dr. #7 actually called me himself with a few questions regarding the ultrasound request. Even though he'd never performed an ultrasound to locate cysts, he was willing to ask his imaging technician to make an attempt.

I returned to his office for the test the next day. Once the imaging tech began the ultrasound, she found the cysts quickly and easily. When I saw Dr. #7 immediately following that ultrasound he told me, "I really don't know what to do about this. I think I should just send you back to Dr. Goldstein."

I know, I know–another red flag. Why, oh why, didn't I heed the warnings? I should have walked out and booked a ticket to San Diego that instant. Instead, I opened my mouth and mentioned that the right cyst was much more noticeable than it was during the previous exam. He agreed to take another look and had no trouble finding the problem spot.

He still didn't believe it was caused by the Bartholin's gland, but he was confident about treatment: A "simple" office procedure. So, against my better judgment, Alan and I returned to his office the next day for treatment.

TIME FOR TREATMENT

The treatment really was simple. Once the tissue was numb the actual procedure took less than five minutes. When he finished, he told us everything went as planned. He said he used a couple of dissolvable sutures and that there would be slight bleeding, the numbing medication would last a few hours (yeah, right), and to return to his office in a week or two for a check-up.

As we stood waiting to make my next appointment and sign paperwork, I was already beginning to experience pain. Twice I almost turned around to tell the nurse or Dr. #7, but I didn't. I thought a little ibuprofen would knock out the pain.

Alan returned to work and my mother-in-law (who had waited with our kids) drove us home. I became increasingly uncomfortable as time passed. When we stopped for lunch, I called Dr. #7's nurse to ask about pain medicine. She didn't answer so I left a voicemail. I decided to visit the closest drugstore for ibuprofen and acetaminophen. I made it to the back of the store and found the painkillers, but by that point I hurt so badly I was not sure I would make it to the cashier. Somehow, I made it to the front of the store. By then my pain had increased to at least a 7 out of 10 and all I wanted to do was ingest those meds and lie flat.

During the remainder of the 20-minute drive home my pain continued to intensify. The nurse had yet to return my call. I should have gone back to the doctor's office at that point, but I didn't.

Then, I had a lightbulb moment; I decided to call Dr. G. Even though he was 1500 miles away, I was certain he would know what to do. Because my kids were in the car, I tried to be calm as I spoke with Alex at SDSM. "I really need to speak with Dr. G–ASAP," I said anxiously. She knew me well so I'm certain she sensed the urgency and pain in my voice. She agreed to have him call me.

About that time, I had a brief moment of relief. I remember it felt like maybe I had a blood clot and it passed, relieving the pressure. Whatever it was, I was thankful to be able to catch a breath.

Finally, Dr. #7's nurse returned my call. I told her I was in extreme pain and asked about the possibility of serious complications. She dismissed the likelihood of anything critical and offered to call the pharmacy with a prescription for pain medication. While we were talking, Dr. G called. It took 90-plus minutes for the local nurse to return my call, and less than five minutes for one of the most skilled sexual medicine doctors in the world to call. Let that sink in.

I quickly dropped the call with her to answer Dr. G's call. He was at a bit of a loss being so far away and not knowing exactly what Dr. #7 had done, but he suggested baths and ice, had his staff call in a script for pain meds, and insisted I keep him updated.

Once we finally made it home, my mother-in-law took my kids to her house and I hurried to the bath. What I found when I undressed to get in the water sent me into panic mode. My right labia was ginormous–which explained the terrible pain. It was also deep purple, nearly black in appearance. I immediately snapped a picture and sent it to Dr. G.

I eased into the warm bath water, hoping it would feel as soothing as it had following my vestibulectomy.

Dr. G responded quickly. He concluded from the photos that Dr. #7 must have had bleeding with the procedure, and suggested I continue rotating between ice and baths. Though I was still in pain, his explanation provided a bit of relief. He assured me I was not going to die. Unless, of course, I died from the pain.

Two and a half hours had passed since the "simple" procedure. The warm bath did not reduce my pain, so I grabbed an ice pack and laid flat on the couch. Shortly after, the pain became so great I could not even produce tears. I could scream and that was about it. It was a good thing we lived in the middle of 140 acres, otherwise I am certain a neighbor would have called 911. On second thought, EMTs would have been helpful, because I was just about ready to find a knife and stab the site–anything to relieve the excruciating pain.

Alan was still 45 minutes away at work so I asked him to head home. Remember, this was happening on a Friday, and come to find out Dr. #7's office closed early on Fridays. So when I tried to call their office again, I heard a recording about how to reach the doctor on call. By that point I couldn't speak. I managed to mutter a few words to Alan - something to the dramatic effect of "find out how to talk to someone who knows what we should do."

A few minutes later, their doctor-on-call called me. I remember saying, "I'm tough, I've had all these surgeries, but I can't take this!" To which he replied, "Well come on up to the ER girl, we'll take care of you!"

GET ME TO THE ER

Getting to the ER was much easier said than done because I had to wait 30 minutes for Alan to get home before we could make the 45-minute drive. Somehow I survived that half-hour. Alan made it home, we grabbed my pain meds, and headed to the ER. I remember hoping we would be pulled over by a highway patrolman who could then take me to the ER at 120 mph instead of 75 mph.

Luckily, when we were about 10 minutes from the hospital, my pain decreased significantly. I don't know if that was due to pain meds or prayer, but I was grateful to be able to breathe again. Once we found the ER entrance and parked Alan left to find a wheel chair.

I really felt sorry for Alan. This was only our third trip to the ER after 10 years of marriage, but all three of those situations were traumatic.

Alan returned with paperwork to get the ball rolling. Between my irrational thinking and honest personality, instead of circling 10/10 on the pain scale I only circled 3/10. As I said, the pain let up about the time we got there. If there ever is a next time for me or any family or friends, I will not hesitate to circle that 10, because less than 10 minutes later the excruciating pain returned. Lesson learned.

Alan took the paperwork to the receptionist and returned with a wheelchair. When we entered the waiting room it was packed. I began to panic at the thought of having to sit and wait. I literally could not sit upright more than a couple of minutes – gravity was my enemy.

From my earlier phone conversation with the doctor-on-call, I was under the impression he would meet us in the ER. My assumption was incorrect.

My pain quickly began to escalate once again. I literally feared my labia would burst at any moment. I had to lie down. I spied a dark, somewhat empty room and instructed

Alan to push me toward it so I could crawl to the floor. Yes, I said floor. *The floor of a hospital emergency room*. Can you say disgusting? I couldn't have cared less about germs as I lay there holding my underwear away from my vagina, trying not to scream like a banshee.

After what felt like an eternity, a nurse came in to inquire about our situation. The conversation went like this:

> Nurse: "I'm sorry honey, but we can't have you lying in here on the floor."
> In my head: "Well okay, then get me a bed!"
> Nurse: "We have to get you in a wheelchair."
> Me: "I can't sit in a wheelchair."
> Nurse: "We can get a pillow."
> In my head: "NO. A freaking pillow will not help! I have a baseball growing in my vagina and I am about to lose my ability to hold myself together, so it would be in your best interest to understand that sooner rather than later."
> Me: "Alan, show him the picture on my phone!"

I kept thinking, "If someone could at least SEE what is happening they will help me."

Turns out the nurse was part of the triage team, so he quickly helped me to a triage unit where my blood pressure reading proved I was legitimately in severe pain. In less than a minute they had me on a bed, in a room, starting an IV. I begged them to take off my pants. Yes, seriously. Since I could barely speak and was nearly hyperventilating, the nurses gathered my history from Alan. I told each new person who entered the room, "Just raise the sheet and look at what is happening." Pain trumps modesty. They would look and quickly respond with, "Oh, I'm so sorry." It took close to 30 minutes for the morphine to make a dent in my pain, but my mind was at ease sooner than that since I knew pain relief was near.

From that point on, the night was like a whirlwind. Thankfully, I had a compassionate, knowledgeable ER doctor who had experience treating Bartholin's cysts. He determined that for unknown reasons I had quite a bit of bleeding after that morning's procedure and the blood became trapped, forming a hematoma.

His recommendation was to do nothing and send me home with pain medication. Wait. Hold up. During the commotion someone had mentioned the hematoma could rupture from the pressure and now they wanted me to go home? Only minutes earlier I had removed my wedding ring and handed it to Alan, fully expecting to be rushed to an operating room. I told Alan I was not leaving. They would at least have to check me into the hospital for the night.

Sometime during that discussion, Dr. G called again. Hearing his voice eased my nerves, until he told me, "This is a definite setback in the process to being pain-free, I will be with you every step of the way, but it will take a while to get past this roadblock."

I began to cry again so I handed the phone to Alan. To my astonishment, Dr. G agreed with the ER doctor's recommendation to do nothing. About the time it became apparent they were serious about kicking me out, my pain escalated. I received one last dose of morphine and a fresh ice pack. Somehow I managed to get my clothes back on and get in our car.

As we left the ER I sent Dr. G an update …

> *"Thank you for giving us hope. It definitely isn't fun. But I am thanking God this didn't happen on an airplane, it's not cancer or something terminal I'm fighting, we have you for support even with so many miles in between, we had family and friends to help with kids and pray for us, and most importantly this wasn't one of our precious kiddos in such horrific pain ... we got this!"*

Dr. G's response ...

> *"You will heal and we will see what has to be done going forward."*

ON THE HEALING ROAD AGAIN

Recovering from that setback was tougher than recovering after the vestibulectomy. Anytime I stood, blood flowed to the area causing extreme pain. I could barely walk. Due to the swelling, I could not wear anything from the waist down for two weeks. The couple of times I did have to leave our house I was barely able to tolerate a pair of Alan's boxers under a sweatshirt dress.

The following Monday morning Dr. #7 called. He knew nothing about my complications until he returned to work that day. He was shocked and sympathetic. He asked if I could visit his office that afternoon. Before he called, I had every intention to never see him again. But once he called, I think I just wanted him to SEE what happened. I wasn't sure Alan could be civil toward that doctor, so I had a friend take me to the appointment. Walking into his office was no small feat–it was both a physical and a mental challenge–but I succeeded.

Needless to say, the doctor was absolutely astonished by what he saw. He said that when he heard what happened he realized I was one of "those" patients. The "if it can go wrong it will" type. I had tried to warn him, but a picture is worth a thousand words.

Four weeks after the "simple-procedure-turned-nightmare" took place, I made my last visit to Dr. #7. By that appointment my vagina no longer looked like it should be part of a science fiction movie. A large portion of the blood that formed the hematoma had re-liquified and drained through the original incision. During that final visit, the doctor was able to gently press around the area and release the majority of the remaining blood. I was thrilled as I stood up and was able to feel the difference. I couldn't wait to wear pants again.

A week later, after a one-month hiatus, I returned to PT. I was understandably apprehensive after the previous month's events, but Becky was extremely careful to avoid aggravating the trauma area. She worked on my exterior muscles to make up some of the ground I'd lost.

PAIN-FREE AT LAST

Nearly a month after resuming physical therapy–two months post-hematoma and seven months post-vestibulectomy–something incredible happened. We discovered a position in which we could achieve pain-free intercourse. One in which there was zero pressure on the tender area. Not only did the sex feel great, but I also felt a weight being lifted from my shoulders. We felt like throwing a party. We felt like blasting Facebook. We felt like calling Dr. G. Of course, we did none of those things, but we remained elated.

JUST KIDDING

I would like to tell you life was only roses from then on; that there was no more pain and we acted like newlyweds, forgetting the heartache of those first 10 years. However, that would be a lie, and I vowed to be honest and open with you.

The truth is, for lots of women that is the case. Once they find a great doctor and the right treatment, they live a pain-free life without setbacks. I truly believe if I'd had the correct treatment from the get-go, I could have been one of those women.

For me, though, it took a few more years of ups and downs to get to that point. If, as you read this book, you feel like you are on the world's longest roller coaster ride–my mission was accomplished. That means I adequately conveyed what our journey felt like.

During the next three years my cysts recurred multiple times. The problem, at least on one side, was that tissue kept covering the opening of the duct, leaving no exit for the fluid produced by that Bartholin's gland, and ultimately forming a painful blister. There were times I would be in so much pain I would have Alan stab the blister with a needle so the fluid could drain and relieve my pain. Even after everything we'd been through that was a new level in our relationship. Each time after the fluid drained, I was left with tender tissue in its wake; meaning intercourse was painful for a few weeks.

Traditional doctors agreed, and still do, that the best treatment for a recurring cyst was to remove the entire Bartholin's gland. While the treatment seemed logical, I was uncomfortable with the risk-to- benefit ratio. The Bartholin's gland is located close to both a major artery and a major nerve. In addition, my sexual medicine expert, Dr. G, pointed out that the gland functioned really well–meaning it pro-

Bartholin's Cyst Marsupialization

Marsupialization is the surgical technique of cutting a slit into an abscess or cyst and suturing the edges of the slit to form a continuous surface from the exterior surface to the interior surface of the cyst or abscess. Sutured in this fashion, the site remains open and can drain freely. This technique is used to treat a cyst or abscess when a single draining would not be effective and complete removal of the surrounding structure would not be desirable.[3]

duced lots of fluid–and it would be a shame to remove such a well-functioning source of lubrication.

Since neither Dr. G nor Alan and I are traditional thinkers, we opted for less invasive approaches. So, during the next two years we experimented with treatments including anti-inflammatory smoothies, essential oils, two trips to San Diego for in-office procedures and two cyst marsupialization's under general anesthesia. We pushed the boundaries. We tried new tricks. Finally, after the second trip to the operating room (that time in Oklahoma–read more about my discovery of a local "Dr. G" in Chapter 10), success was ours. It was a long, winding road, the end of which we were all shocked and thrilled to reach.

After 13 years of ups, downs, joys and heartaches, we truly understood the following words penned by Maryann Radmacher:

Courage doesn't always roar. Sometimes courage
is the quiet voice at the end of the day saying
'I will try again tomorrow.'

9

Mind Over Matter

Our afflictions are not imposed by the Divine. Rather, they lead us to the Divine more often than our joys do. Do not resist the bitter pills in your life; know that they will lead you to a greater awareness.

Bernie Siegel, MD

That was the easy part.

Yes, you read that right. After all the doctors, questions, hospitals, Internet searches, stress, long nights, long days, books, supplements, therapies, essential oils, hopes, disappointments, progress, and setbacks; after working so hard to diagnose and heal the physical, I was left with the aftermath: Emotions. More than 10 years' worth of emotions that I had stuffed deep inside my heart; as well as, walls of numbness I'd built subconsciously, brick by brick, in an effort to shield myself from both the physical and the emotional pain.

EARLY ON

During the first few years after we wed, I felt like a failure as a woman. Like my body would not let us experience the great pleasure God intended, nor would it let me be the help-meet my husband so desperately wanted and needed. Alan would optimistically encourage me, saying, "Let's just try (intercourse), maybe it won't hurt this time." And I would think, "How would it not hurt?! Nothing has changed. It is going to hurt. It always has and this time will be no different."

I loved my husband tremendously and longed for that missing intimate connection, so I would mentally dig down until I found a sliver of hope, we would try again, and once more there would be physical pain. Even worse than the physical pain, though, was the chronic emotional pain of disappointment and loss.

In those times, had I asked, most experts would have told me to "think positive" and "control your mental chatter." I did buy the theory that "what you think is what you get" and respected the power of the mind-body connection. However, in those moments of vulnerability, fear, and traumatic recollections, changing one's thoughts is a million times easier said than done. Add to that the fact that I knew I had a real, physical problem and it did hurt every time we tried to have intercourse. Positive thinking did not cut it.

As the years progressed, it got to a point where after each painful experience I would lie facing the wall, curled in the fetal position, trying to think of anything other than the reality of the moment, and praying sleep would be instant. I wanted to run far away. I would have done anything to get rid of those feelings of worthlessness, which were magnified by the lack of hope and absence of answers from doctors.

Attempting to avoid the pain, I tried to ignore those negative feelings. I tried to numb the pain. However, those efforts were unsuccessful because, "We can't selectively numb emotion. Numb the dark and you numb the light.[1]"

I thought I was succeeding. I thought I was hiding my feelings from myself and from those around me. I lived under the assumption that I was acting as I always had–with confidence, clarity, compassion, hope, love and zeal for God, love for others, joy, kindness, passion, and optimism - and simply ignoring the sadness, heartache, disappointment, and frustration.

The reality, though, was that I spent so long trying to be tough, strong, positive, and silent about our struggles, that I lost my joy and hope along the way. The result was a change at my core, in my heart.

Instead of numbing my negative emotions, or even numbing all my emotions, I somehow accomplished the opposite: I severed the positive ones. The result was a lack of balance that left me using my emotional energy to produce negative reactions. While I could still get fired up and be passionate, it was not always in a good way. In short, I was angry.

ANGER: A PRIMARY EMOTION

In Dr. David Hanscom's book, *Back In Control*, he discusses his personal journey through chronic pain. He dedicates an entire chapter to what he titles "The Ultimate Modifier–Anger." Hanscom opens that chapter with a sequence of events that cause anger:

1. Circumstance (real or imagined)
2. Blame
3. Victimhood
4. Frustration and Anger

"In this sequence," Hanscom explains, "you blame a person or circumstance for disrupting your sense of well-being, which places you in the role of victim, and you become angry."

How does that apply in cases of sexual dysfunction? Most of us are familiar with Maslow's Hierarchy of Needs and his theory that if a person's 'deficiency needs' (the bottom four levels) are not met, they become anxious.[2] Sexual intimacy falls under the "social," or third, level of Maslow's pyramid. So, when our innate need and desire for sexual intimacy is not met for an extended period of time, no matter the reason, we perceive it as a loss of control and thus anger (anxiety with a chemical kick[3]) likely sets in.

What's interesting about primary emotions is that they are, indeed, primary. What we usually express though, are the secondary emotions. As mentioned above, feelings like *frustration* and *anxiety* are actually rooted in *anger.*

When you study the wheel of emotions, based on the six basic emotions identified by Paul Ekman in 1972[4] (Happiness, Sadness, Disgust, Anger, Fear, and Surprise) you will notice that "Anger" is opposite "Happy." Notice also that there are four primary emotions between the two. Based on

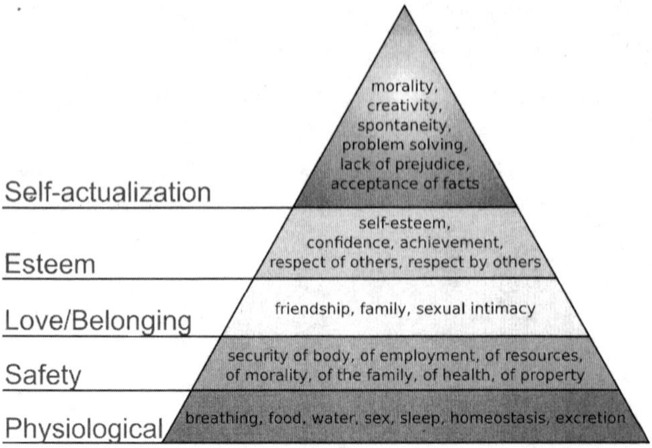

Figure 9.1

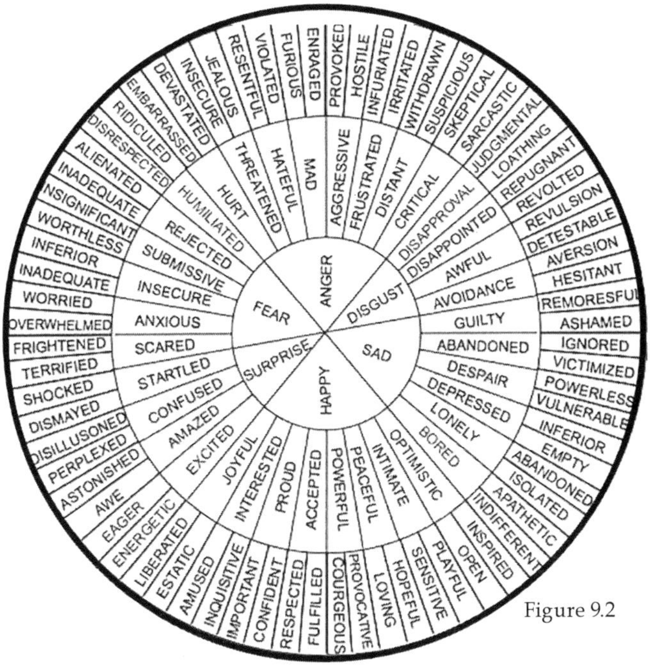

Figure 9.2

my personal experiences and observations, the key to triggering anger lies somewhere in those middle emotions of Sadness, Disgust, Fear, and Surprise.

Looking back, I can track the connection between the emotions I felt on our wedding night and finding myself rife with anger more than 10 years later.

I began our marriage journey confident, optimistic, and eager (Happy/Surprise), only to quickly find myself dismayed, confused, and in despair (Surprise/Sadness). Through the years, with disinterested doctors, failed treatments, and tension from lack of intimacy (more on that later); I began to feel insecure, guilty, and isolated (Fear/Sadness).

The unfortunate reality of sexual pain, in particular, is that it leads to a brutal mental, emotional, and physical spiral. Each painful experience made me less likely to desire sex. Loss of desire eventually led to disinterest altogether. Finally, disinterest became avoidance (Disgust).

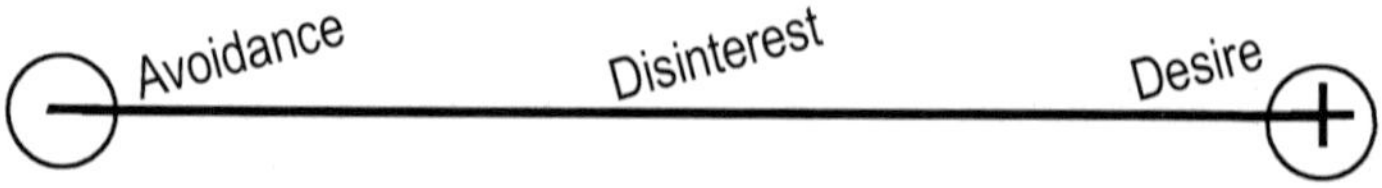

In my simple illustration of desire, I view avoidance as the "negative" end of the spectrum. The point where you want to evade sexual encounters altogether. Disinterest is neutral. Desire, of course, is on the positive end.

All those feelings were bearable, though, while I was experiencing physical pain–because I had something to blame. Something to serve as a distraction. I was the victim. As Goldstein, Goldstein and Pukall point out in *When Sex Hurts*, "Pain was the scapegoat[5]."

However, when the physical pain resolved, and I did not immediately return to the old "me," I was lost. I believed our marriage would instantly mend when we could finally have intercourse, but it didn't. I thought my lack of desire/disinterest/avoidance would magically regress – not so much.

It was at that point I began to feel frustrated, hurt, insecure, distant, and hostile (Anger). That was my breaking point. I'd held on so long, sometimes with only the tip of my finger. But when the chronic emotional pain did not disappear with the physical pain, I lost my endpoint. My hope disappeared along with my faith. My hand slipped and I began to free-fall into the "abyss of anger[6]."

NUMBING VS. AWARENESS

What I did not know at the time, but makes sense, is that my efforts to numb the pain, to avoid facing the feelings, were in vain. Unlike our physical selves, which can continue healing while our pain is numbed, if we try to 'numb' emotional pain, we get a break from the pain … but the "healing is put on pause too[7]."

So, instead of getting rid of those feelings, I'd actually buried them alive. At that point, out of necessity to escape, they were beginning to make themselves known by governing my thoughts, attitude, and emotional reactions[8]. Though I tried to hide my mental implosion from the world, I imagine at times I looked like the utter destruction described here:

> *For a seed to achieve its greatest expression, it must come completely undone. The shell cracks, its insides come out and everything changes. To someone who doesn't understand growth, it would look like complete destruction.*
> Cynthia Occelli

I wrote the following words during that time …

It wasn't pretty. It was ugly. It was difficult. I turned away from God instead of to Him. I chose to live selfishly and in the moment. To become unbalanced and extreme and ungrateful. To not care for my husband and his needs. To let my children stress me out. To get my priorities out of line. But I am ever so thankful, because I have changed. I believe I am on the path to growing into the woman God has wanted me to be. He knew the path I would choose. He placed the right people, the right experiences, the right roadblocks to keep me close enough that I could get back on the path without too much stumbling. He gave me the watering and fertiliz-

ing I needed to change. He was there the whole time. And He will be with me until my last breath. I can choose to hold onto Him or not, but He won't leave (Isaiah 59:1-2). I pray I choose to stay with Him. My eternity depends on it, and my earthly life and family will be a thousand times better for it.

Though at times I doubted God's ways, I did hold on to the belief that somehow, someway, I could change; I could heal.

As Brendon Burchard so confidently states, "I believe in my ability to learn and figure things out. With enough focus, time, effort, and dedication, I believe I can learn to do what must be done and become who I must become to achieve my dreams."

So, I scoured the internet; read books by pioneers Brene Brown, Ruth Haley Barton, Joe Dispenza and the like; reopened my Bible; and found qualified mental health professionals willing to listen and guide me.

As I studied, a common theme emerged: Awareness.

Hanscom defines awareness in *Back in Control* as "seeing the world as it actually is–not your interpretation of it."

Webster's College Dictionary defines it as "knowing or realizing, conscious, informed."

As Hanscom makes clear, positive thinking is the opposite of awareness. Positive thinking causes thought suppression, while awareness connects us to our thoughts and environment[9].

I was willing to admit that my skills were less than ideal when it came to awareness. I also knew I could no longer suppress my thoughts and feelings, so I began to build my awareness muscles. Oddly, the best advice for becoming more aware was to do less. Slowing down was not my style, but I gave it my all.

FEELING THE FEELINGS

One of the hardest things for me, which is probably also the case for the majority of people, is to let myself feel my feelings. I know that sounds redundant and ridiculously simple, but it's true.

I had to learn to be okay with feeling mad, or sad, or hurt, or scared, or frustrated, or questioning why things were happening. I had to retrain my brain to believe that it was, in fact, healthy to feel my feelings. Acknowledging my feelings was the only way I could truly process them and get to the other side. The side where I could react using my rational, conscious mind.

That was quite an adjustment. As I realized after reading Joe Dispenza's *Breaking the Habit of Being Yourself*, for nearly 35 years I lived by habit. Psychologists say that by the time we're in our mid-30s our personality is completely formed. That means we have programmed our subconscious with a set of thoughts, attitudes, behaviors and reactions that run on autopilot. In other words: Habits. From washing our hair to driving down the highway, those habits make up about 95 percent of our mind. Leaving only five percent of our mind to make conscious choices[10].

Dispenza makes a profound observation: When we try to take the place back and "we cease the habitual action, chaos rages between the body and the mind[11]."

My valiant efforts to increase awareness and restore my joy, hope, and confidence, were met with resistance by a lifelong habit of being a champion feeling-stuffer.

I learned that my emotions were a bit like glass lenses. If you've ever worn glasses, or even sunglasses, I bet you can remember a time when you made a quick transition from a warm house out into the cold or vice versa. The result: Instant fog. So much fog that you can't see. Sure, you can take the glasses off, wipe away the condensation, and the lenses will stay clear for a few seconds. But, once you return them to your face, the condensation returns. Eventually, the lenses adjust to the new temperature and the condensation dissipates. Emotions are similar. We can try to hide them or "wipe them off," but they quickly return to cloud our judgment. Only when we truly learn to be still with those feelings, without judgment, and then let them pass, are we truly able to see clearly.

I slowly managed to release the power of anger and allow myself to feel the sadness, hurt, frustration, and guilt I'd carried through the years. The crazy thing, just like so many experts said would be the case, was that as I faced those feelings instead of turning from them, they drifted away. The change was not quick, nor was it easy or painless. As Hanscom points out, awareness is the antithesis of anger[12]. I had a wide chasm to bridge. Eventually, though, as I felt my feelings and learned my triggers, I made my way back to the "Happy" section of the wheel.

Do I still have more to learn? Absolutely. Is it still a struggle to live from a place of awareness and slow my reactions? Yep. Did it fix all my problems? No way. For me, part of learning to live from a space of awareness meant adopting Tony Robbins' CANI philosophy: Constant And Never-ending Improvement. Learning to accept that I am not where I want to be, and because the bar keeps rising, I never will be. As long as I am better today than I was yesterday, that is enough.

MY OTHER HALF

At this point you may be thinking, "That explains a lot about the way you overcame your individual obstacles, but weren't you still married? What was happening in your marriage?"

Those are valid questions. Yes, I was still married and some rough things were happening between Alan and me.

After years of going through the motions and figuring out ways for both of us to achieve some sort of sexual release, our sexual relationship became mechanical. There was no intimacy involved. We weren't making love. We were only increasing hostility toward each other based on what we thought the other wasn't giving.

Naturally, those frustrations carried over into every aspect of our relationship. For him (I get how this is the case) he didn't just want the act from me, he wanted me to want a sexual relationship. While I understood that intellectually, and searched and searched within my mind for a "switch" to flip, I couldn't find it. Trying to please him sexually when I wanted absolutely nothing at all to do with it wasn't exactly a turn-on for either of us.

Alan and I both naively believed that when we resolved the physical pain my desire would return in a snap, our frustrations with each other would disappear, and we would begin to experience the intimacy we both so desperately desired. When that did not happen, we were both equally devastated and lost.

TRUE INTIMACY

As Ed Wheat, MD, explains so well in his incredible book *Intended for Pleasure*:

> Real sexual intimacy links marriage partners with strong strands of caring that are deeply emotional, mental–even spiritual–and also intensely physical; thus closeness does not occur only at times of intercourse …. Developing real sexual

> intimacy carries a couple safely through the traditionally dangerous water of the first several years of marriage ... But the other side of the coin is also true. Because sexual intimacy is so important as a constructive, integrative force, when it is disappointing or absent altogether, it has an enormous potential for disruption of the marriage.[13]

Even after 12 years of marriage, we were unaware that sex and intimacy were not synonymous. We didn't realize how everything that happened in our marriage had an effect on our lovemaking.

Unfortunately, in those early years we were unable to develop the sexual intimacy that Wheat describes. As the years progressed, we began to feel the "potential for disruption."

While I would love to tell you we quickly identified our issues and found ways to mend our wounds, that wasn't the case. We were both so jaded that our patience for each other and will to fight began to waiver.

I remember one time Alan asked a friend to counsel us. During that session, our friend suggested Alan and I read the Bible and pray together nightly and spend more time together as a couple. While the intellectual part of me knew how beneficial that could be, the emotional side screamed, "How in the world can we do that? I can't get him to talk about anything!" Praying together is such an intimate action, and I knew it would bring to light the fact that not only was I unhappy with my husband and myself, I was also unhappy with God. It felt as if He had abandoned me. Though I had an unjustified and ungrateful attitude, my feelings were very real.

I began to wonder if our relationship was worth fighting for. We had worked and worked, but I felt like Alan wasn't listening, and he felt like I wasn't trying. We knew we made vows to each other and to God–for better or for worse, in sickness and in health–but the emotional pain and struggle was so great that at times those words seemed impossible to uphold. I was tired and scared; mentally and emotionally exhausted. I didn't feel like I had anything left to give. That was a scary place.

SEEKING ANSWERS

Honestly, had we not had kids, I am not sure how things would have played out. While I didn't have a clue how to save our marriage, I did know I did know I needed to find a way for the sake of our three amazing kiddos. I was aware that I could not give them what I didn't have. I also realized the only way our children would choose marriages full of love and forgiveness was if we demonstrated those characteristics to them through our marriage.

I began to wonder if, after all the physical and emotional trauma, I had developed a form of post-traumatic stress disorder (PTSD). I thought that maybe, just maybe, if I could rewire my brain to stop thinking of intercourse as painful, then I would desire it again and all our marital troubles would resolve. It sounded simple enough. If I could want sex, and if it could be pain-free, all would be well.

Alan actually agreed with my theory. So, with PTSD as a self-diagnosis we both searched for something that might help. I'd been through hours of "talk therapy" with a handful of counselors. While I am thankful for those sessions, and am a better person because of every hour spent, I knew that was not the answer. It just so happened, as we were searching, I met a therapist who specialized in EMDR (eye movement desensitization reprocessing)–a fairly new therapy commonly used as a treatment modality for PTSD. She also mentioned that she worked often with mothers who had lost children. Coincidence? I think not. As He had done so many times before, God brought the perfect person into my life at the perfect time. So, I began EMDR therapy.

The same week that I found the EMDR option, Alan discovered hypnotherapy. It seemed we were grasping at straws, but as usual I was open to trying just about anything. In addition, psychology had always fascinated me; I was intrigued to learn if and how hypnotherapy could work for me, so I also scheduled a hypnotherapy consultation and subsequent session.

Eye Movement Desensitization Reprocessing

EMDR (Eye Movement Desensitization Reprocessing) is a therapy method originally developed to treat post-traumatic stress disorder in combat veterans. It is now used to treat a variety of conditions in addition to the effects of trauma. Those conditions include panic attacks, complicated grief, phobias, eating disorders, chronic pain, performance anxiety, abuse and others. It uses rapid eye movement, sounds or vibrations to trigger the brain to reprocess memories. Reprocessing memories allows the release and transformation of negative thoughts and painful emotions related to the memory. The memory transforms from a painful/traumatic memory to an ordinary one. EMDR was developed in the 1980s by Dr. Francine Shapiro, PhD. It is recognized as an effective treatment method by the American Psychiatric Association, the International Society for Traumatic Stress Studies, the World Health Organization, the Department of Defense and the U.S. Department of Veterans Affairs, among others.

Contribution by Susan Bachmann, LPC, NCC
Family Therapy and Renewal Center

Hypnotherapy

Hypnotherapy makes use of a natural and relaxed state of mind that most people experience regularly. A state of relaxation and concentration facilitates accessibility to deeper parts of the mind and heightens a subject's receptivity to suggestion. Hypnotherapy promotes reduction of stress, anxiety, fears, and phobias; release of emotional attachments; pain management; grief release; acceptance of change; improved sleep; and much more. It is not brainwashing, and a hypnotherapist cannot make a person do anything he or she doesn't want to do. One's memory and faculties are fully aware during hypnosis. Hypnotherapy is safe and accepted by progressive medicine and science as a helpful treatment tool for many conditions, including those mentioned above.

Browning Clinical Hypnotherapy

I found both therapies to be extremely beneficial, with quite a few similarities. I can only speak from my experience, but for me, they were both great diagnostic tools.

I typically have a lot of "noise" in my mind. I can change the topic of conversation 10 times in a minute. My noisy mind, combined with my tendency to suppress emotions and my human nature to avoid pain, made finding the root cause of my emotional trauma quite a challenge.

EMDR and hypnotherapy both helped me navigate through my conscious mind and tap into my subconscious. They both aided my efforts to live from a place of awareness. I left the hypnotherapy sessions in a less anxious, more clear state of mind. I often left EMDR sessions thinking, "How do those pieces fit together?" Both were positive experiences that lead to helpful discoveries, including these two epiphanies:

1. There was a psychosomatic component to the recurrence of my cyst. Every time I discussed the pain or the struggles in our relationship, the cyst returned. At first, I thought it was coincidence, but after it happened three or four times I could not ignore the connection. That's not to say the pain was only "in my head" the entire 13 years. That was not the case at all. But there was definitely a psychological component causing a physical manifestation.

2. I discovered that underneath the anger, sadness, and disappointment I had worked so hard to sort through, there was a sincere fear that maybe my sexual dysfunction was not the only "dysfunction" in our relationship. What if, when my pain was gone entirely, we still had problems? And what if those problems were more than either of us could handle? I had learned how to release my own emotional pain, but what would happen if the focus shifted from the physical pain in our relationship to a pain we were not willing to face as a couple?

From the outside looking in, these epiphanies made complete sense. While it may not be widely accepted, there is sufficient evidence to prove that not only do our thoughts create our reality[14], they also alter the chemical composition and behavior of our cells[15]. For example, think of the physical reactions that typically occur when a person prepares for a job interview: Sweaty palms, nausea, dry mouth, etc.

In addition, based on the lack of care we had given our relationship during those first 12 years–aggravated by our sub-par communication skills–my fear of wide-spread relationship dysfunction was logical. At the same time, I couldn't let the fear of not knowing the outcome stop me from trying. I had to find the courage to face the uncertainty.

I remember putting my newfound awareness to work one night when I felt like I was at my wits end and ready to throw in the towel. I was able to vocalize my feelings and tell Alan, "I am tired of getting the leftovers. I am exhausted and don't have anything left to give. I don't know what else to do for us." That night, for the first time in years, the emotional floodgates opened and the tears I'd fought so hard to hold back through the years flowed down my cheeks. My guard came down. I ended up sobbing in Alan's arms, which was oddly refreshing. I was finally able to feel and express my emotions again. Coincidentally, that breakdown - or breakthrough - occurred on our wedding anniversary and in that moment I realized my deepest desire hadn't changed much through the years:

In the end, we all just want someone who chooses us, over everyone else, under any circumstances.
Anonymous

NEUROPLASTICITY

After my positive experiences with hypnotherapy and EMDR (both treatments I will utilize when necessary in the future), I found one more "out of the box" treatment modality to help counteract the years of emotional turmoil: Neurofeedback. I honestly don't even remember how I stumbled upon neurofeedback, but I thank God I did.

I believed in the theory of the brain's ability to "rewire" itself through practices like yoga and meditation. In addition, I'd heard of neurofeedback as a treatment for concussions and other traumatic brain injuries (TBIs), so it wasn't much of a leap to imagine neurofeedback could restore cog-

Neurofeedback

Neurofeedback is a non-invasive therapy that trains the brain to self-regulate and normalize. It uses the most foundational therapeutic principle of operant conditioning: positive feedback for desired behaviors. Using this concept, it is possible to create new neuropathways by consistently training brainwave activity to stay within normal, healthy ranges. Neuropathways are naturally formed and reinforced in response to our environment, thoughts, emotions, and injury. These pathways can be normal, functional, and healthy, or they can be abnormal and cause undesirable symptoms and behaviors. Our brains can intentionally and purposefully create new, more desirable neuropathways or 'psychological highways' through consistent training. The more we train a certain neural pathway, the stronger it will become - much like exercising a muscle. Over time, these stronger, healthier pathways become the favored ones, and healthy function becomes the "new norm." For this reason, neurofeedback offers long-lasting and permanent change.

Contribution by Dannelle Newnam, LPC
Oklahoma Neurofeedback Specialists

nitive function in other parts of the brain. I'd recognized for a few years that my brain wasn't working like it had before. I kept thinking, "I wasn't always this way." I felt like my mind could not focus on even the simplest tasks such as making a grocery list. As I began to research neurofeedback as a treatment option for restoring overall brain function, I began to wonder what kind of impact it could have on my emotional health.

After a brief consultation with Dannelle Newnam of Oklahoma Neurofeedback Specialists, I was hooked. The first step of treatment was to perform an EEG (electroencephalogram) to establish a baseline of brainwave activity.

The readings of the initial EEG were then combined with my answers to a set of questionnaires, to assess my overall sense of wellbeing. I was intrigued as I looked through my initial paperwork. My assessment noted poor cognitive efficiency in the areas of attention, verbal processing, and reading comprehension–no surprise there. However, I was a bit surprised by the self-dimensional findings that showed abnormal results in areas of depression, anxiety, impulsivity, assertiveness, and perfectionism.

As I stepped back to consider the truth of those results, they began to make sense. They were all after-effects of more than 13 years of chronic emotional turmoil. The good news was, after 20 sessions of neurofeedback, my final EEG showed a 33 percent improvement in brainwave activity. Not only that, but the markers on the self-dimensional assessment showed a noticeable improvement. Finally, and most importantly, I felt like I could focus my mind and live from a proactive instead of reactive state once again. As I had hoped, my results significantly improved our marriage.

WHAT HAPPENED, HAPPENED

I must admit, this chapter was the hardest for me to write. Not only was it distressing to live the journey I chronicled in these pages, it was also uncomfortable to relive. In fact, even as it is ready for print, I am still nervous about letting others see this part of me. Through the years I shared pieces of this part of my life with others, but never did I put all the pieces together to show anyone the whole picture.

I feel like some will read this chapter, consider me crazy, and wonder why I didn't just "pull myself together." Sometimes I wondered that myself. But I did my best with the resources I had. It wasn't easy to admit I needed help, nor was it easy to ask for help. It still isn't easy to share my story. However, each step of the way I did what I needed to do to get where I wanted to be, and for that I am grateful. As for the crazy, well I can't deny that completely since my laptop's wallpaper is Apple's famous commercial narrative, "Here's to the Crazy Ones."

I feel others will read this chapter and think of all the things I should have done differently. While I am the first to admit I am far from perfect and could have made some wiser, less selfish choices, I know that I cannot change the past. What happened, happened. And as Jim Rohn says, "It's not what happens, it's what you do."

What Alan and I both have and will choose to do, is to learn from our mistakes and use the strength we gained from our trials to be our best–for each other, for our children, for our friends, for our fellow man, and for God.

She could never go back and make some of the details pretty. All she could do was move forward and make the whole beautiful.
Terri St. Cloud

Section Three:

to Empower

The question is not, will there be difficulties
and threats to our existence,
but how will we deal with them and
what can we learn from them.
How can they become blessings to society,
as a life-threatening disease is to an
individual, by teaching us about
the meaning of our life and existence?
Bernie Siegel, M.D.

10

Paying it Forward

Where you're wounded, you're gifted.
Carl Jung

Never in my wildest dreams would I have imagined writing a book that had anything to do with sexual dysfunction, speaking in front of a group about my struggles with sexual pain, or being quoted in a *New York Times* article about my lack of sexual desire. Yet, I have done all those and more. Somewhere along our journey, as I learned just how little doctors are taught about women's sexual dysfunction, the vast number of women affected by some sort of sexual pain, and the lack of support and resources available to us, I decided to be part of the solution. While filling that role wasn't always easy, it was (and still is) always worth it.

IT BEGAN WITH TALK THERAPY

Playing the hand Alan and I were dealt was hard. Playing that hand on our own was even harder. Granted, we both could have shared our struggles with others sooner than we did. However, between our independent, introverted personalities and a general lack of awareness concerning the commonality of sexual dysfunction, Alan and I both chose to keep our tribulations quiet. Sex was not exactly a topic about which we would ask for guidance from Facebook friends–or any friends for that matter.

So, when Dr. G first suggested I write about our experience in the forums of his website (http://sexualmed.org) I immediately said, "No way! Not for me." He persisted; reminding me of the therapeutic benefits of talk therapy. Eventually I agreed and I am certainly glad I did.

I began to chronicle our journey post-op while I was still taking prescription pain medication, which made it a little easier to be honest and open in my writing; maybe not clear or coherent, but honest and open. As I wrote, I slowly uncovered my lost love for writing. Before I had children, writing was a pillar of my identity. Even though the style of writing I used for the forum was much different than the journalistic-style to which I was accustomed, it renewed my passion nonetheless.

Of course, you could not have convinced me then that four short years later I would pull from those thoughts to publish my first book, but here it is. God definitely has a unique way of using everyday opportunities as stair steps to bigger things in our lives.

PROSPECTIVE PATIENTS

Before I had both my VAT and my vestibulectomy, Dr. G sent me a list of contact information for women who had been through each procedure. Emailing and speaking by phone with some of those ladies made my fears about the procedures subside. Not only were the women satisfied with their decisions to undergo the procedures, they also had complete confidence in Dr. G.

So, when it came my turn to pay it forward and do the same for other women, I was happy to oblige. I found, as I spoke with ladies on the path before and after me, that it was not nearly as uncomfortable to discuss such personal issues with those women. Not only because we shared a common pain, but because we also shared a common glimmer of hope. We had Dr. G and we had each other. We were truly blessed.

NATIONAL VULVODYNIA ASSOCIATION*

After I began sharing with women who were already on a similar path, Dr. G encouraged me to step-up my support role and serve as a support leader for the NVA–an organization of which I was a five-year member. I must admit I was a bit hesitant, but once I spoke with the director of support services for the NVA, I was game. As a support leader, I communicate by email or phone with members who need a listening ear or encouragement to keep going.

Serving the members of the NVA remains bittersweet. I still feel awkward emailing new members. It sounds strange to say, "I am glad you joined our group," because I am not glad they have vulvodynia. I am genuinely glad, however, that they found the courage to look for answers and reach out for help. I pray as I serve the members to whom I am assigned that I can show them hope, light, and love; qualities that do not come from me but from my Almighty God.

Take joy in sharing positive energy with others.
It's a rough road for all, so give the sunlight.
Brendon Burchard

*The NVA is a non-profit organization that strives to "improve women's health through education, research, support and advocacy." Find out more at www.nva.org.

Note: A portion of the proceeds from the sale of this book will be donated to the NVA.

NURSE PRACTITIONERS IN WOMEN'S HEALTH*

In the summer of 2014 I was invited to the great state of Texas to speak at the inaugural Women's Sexual Health Course for Nurse Practitioners. That was shortly after my autumn surgery in California and spring visit to the emergency room in Oklahoma. When Catherine Gagnon, NP at SDSM, emailed me inquiring about my willingness to make the four-hour trip and speak during one of the break-out sessions with Dr. G, I was hesitant. Do you see a trend here? Hesitant to write, hesitant to lead, hesitant to speak–God definitely used the aforementioned opportunities to stretch my comfort zone. I told her I would think about it. A couple of days later, Dr. G called asking the same question. How could I refuse after everything he had done for me? So, I agreed.

The entire month between making the commitment and speaking in Dallas, I was a basket case. It had been nearly seven years since I had done any sort of public speaking, and I had never talked to an audience of more than one about such a personal topic. Add to that, the only real details I received about the event were the location, time, and that we would be sharing our story to a group of either 50 or 200. Zero pressure.

I was a stressed-out mess by the time that weekend arrived. Being the ever-steady-force-of-calm he always is, Alan attempted to help me pull myself together. My nerves were just about shot by the time we arrived at the conference hotel. However, once we found Dr. G and his beautiful wife, Sue, my butterflies nearly disappeared.

Our final plan was to speak four consecutive times, as NPs rotated through our break-out session. Five minutes into speaking to the first group, I was at ease. I would share a piece of our story, then Dr. G would allow the NPs "diagnose" me. He also gave the time to ask questions to help in their diagnoses. By the time we finished speaking to the second group, I felt like I was in my element. It felt great to share our story with practitioners who were eager to learn from our experience so they could return home to provide better care to their own patients.

I share that story, and the others in this chapter, not to highlight a single thing about myself, but to encourage you to push your limits and trust God. Within a few short hours that evening, I experienced a drastic improvement in my emotional state and level of confidence. I went from feeling scared to death and nearly throwing up, to feeling both successful and sad when our last session ended. I am forever grateful for that opportunity to expand my comfort zone.

What if I fall?
Oh, but my darling, what if you fly?
Erin Hanson

*The mission of the National Association of Nurse Practitioners in Women's Health is to ensure the provision of quality primary and specialty healthcare to women of all ages by women's health and women's health focused nurse practitioners. For more information visit www.npwh.org.

COFFEE DATE GROUP

Nearly a year after I volunteered to be an NVA support leader, I received an exciting member assignment–my very first Oklahoma member. Around the same time, yet another Oklahoma woman contacted me after finding my email address online. I corresponded with each of the ladies by email for a few months before we all three agreed we would like to meet for coffee to put faces with names.

At that point, even I had not sat face-to-face with a fellow patient. We enjoyed our time together and continued to meet periodically during the next year. The camaraderie we shared and encouragement we gained from our coffee dates propelled us to consider expanding our group. I knew two of my fellow leaders on the West Coast organized monthly NVA meetings, so I knew it was doable. Those leaders emailed me copies of their agendas, sign-in sheets, rules, dos and don'ts–everything needed to get the ball rolling. The only thing stopping us was us.

FLIBANSERIN (ADDYI)

The fall of 2015 was a pivotal time for women's health. The FDA finally approved a game-changer for women with Hypoactive Sexual Desire Disorder (HSDD): Flibanserin, also known as Addyi. Supporters of the drug termed it the "little pink pill;" opponents claimed an inadequate risk-to-benefit ratio and continued fighting against it long after the approval.

Because I had great results with flibanserin shortly after it became available to the public, Dr. G asked if I would be willing to speak with reporters composing articles about it. Of course, I agreed.

I was anxious about the interviews, the way the reporters might write their articles, and who would read my quotes. Much to my relief, my fears subsided when I read their final news pieces. Here is an excerpt from the CNN story[1]:

"I love my husband and I believe God created emotional and sexual intimacy as key components of marriage. So, we had sex, usually a couple of times a week. And while I was willing, part of me dreaded it. Every time." Cole said she started taking Addyi in November, and within six weeks felt a difference. "I was amazed," she wrote. "I actually enjoyed being intimate and for the first time in a long time felt that connection with Alan." She said for her it wasn't about increasing the quantity of sex she was having, but rather the quality. "What [Addyi] does is give just enough support so I can think about that part of our relationship with anticipation of pleasure rather than anxiety," she wrote. She understands Addyi can have side effects, but said women should be able to choose to take it just as men choose to take Viagra despite its side effects. "I should be able to choose whether the side effects are worth the benefit."

Every effort I made to break the silence surrounding women's sexual dysfunction was way out of my "box." Yet, each step of the way, encouraging emails like the one below fueled my passion for the cause.

"Hi Dr. Goldstein – I just saw the NY Times article about flibanserin yesterday. What a great article! I have to say how appreciative I am of your patient for her courage to discuss the issue. I know you assured me that other women my age were suffering through this, but it was wonderfully eye opening to hear her story and know that I am not the only one."

PUBLIC SUPPORT GROUP

You know how I said the only thing preventing our coffee group from "going public" was us? Well, God helped us get out of our own way. One of the ladies started seeing a local pelvic floor PT, Megan Warner. During one of her appointments she mentioned our idea to Megan, who immediately jumped on board and volunteered to host meetings in her clinic.

Since we were completely without excuse, we set a date and began to advertise that first meeting. I shared the news with my former PT, Becky Wilcox, who actively joined forces by inviting patients and colleagues. We had nine attendees the night of our inaugural event, each of whom engaged openly in conversation and expressed interest in future meetings.

Looking around the circle of women that evening, I kept thinking, "We did it. We finally made this happen."

TULSA WOMEN'S HEALTH ALLIANCE*

When I decided to support women and aid in breaking the silence surrounding female sexual dysfunction, I had no idea where that decision would lead. There was no path to follow–which was actually fine by me. My entire life I had lived by Ralph Waldo Emerson's words, "Do not go where the path may lead, go instead where there is no path and leave a trail." Over the years, as I said "yes" to the opportunities mentioned above, my passion and mission for helping women continued to grow.

The series of events that unfolded after our first public meeting were almost too good to be true. We held our second meeting five months after the first meeting. Immediately after that second meeting, connections began falling into place. Becky mentioned a local gynecologist, Dr. Corey Babb, who specialized in women's sexual health. I was eager to network by reaching out to others with similar interests, so I immediately sent him an email to set up a time to discuss his focus and experience. I will admit I was a bit skeptical, having searched 12 years without luck for a local doctor with more than basic training in the field of gynecology.

Much to my astonishment, Dr. Babb was the real deal. He knew about the NVA and knew of Dr. Goldstein. He was registered to attend the fall course of the International Society for the Study of Women's Sexual Health. He even knew of and prescribed flibanserin to applicable patients. Most importantly, after only five minutes of conversation, I knew he grasped the complexity of women's sexuality and took a holistic approach to caring for his patients with compassion. I was shocked and excited to add him to our network. I was especially ecstatic when he agreed to speak at our next meeting.

By the third meeting we recruited two more PTs, two additional mental health therapists and a pharmacist–all with a shared passion for women's health–bringing the total count to 10 providers. At that point, we realized it was time to create a plan to combine our forces to reach women in Tulsa and the surrounding communities. We scheduled a brainstorming session before our next meeting; during that session the Tulsa Women's Health Alliance was born.

Our group has big goals to help women right here at home, and I have no doubt we have the passion and determination to achieve those goals.

*The TWHA's mission is to increase awareness while supporting, educating, and empowering women suffering with pelvic pain and the struggles associated with that pain. For more information visit

www.tulsawomenshealthalliance.com.

WHAT'S YOUR ROLE?

If, as you read through this chapter you thought, "I want to help with this mission!" Great. The more people working to banish the stigma of sexual pain the better. Listed below are a few ways patients can help:

1. Join and/or donate to organizations such as the National Vulvodynia Association to help fund research.
2. Write your story and share it where you feel comfortable – in forums, social media groups, blogs, etc.
3. If you haven't already, share your story with those in your circle who will lend a supportive, listening ear.
4. Volunteer for appropriate clinical trials.
5. Create your own outreach. The sky is the limit.

If, as you read through this chapter you thought, "Increasing awareness about sexual pain is not my passion, but 'X' is." Great. I encourage you to go out and make a difference in the area about which you are passionate.

In the words of Howard Thurman: "Don't ask yourself what the world needs. Ask yourself what makes you come alive and then go do that. Because what the world needs is people who have come alive."

What makes you come alive? What strengths and talents did God place in you that are ready to escape the bonds of fear and doubt to make a wave of change in our world? If you are unsure, spend some time in solitude and prayer. Think through the trials and tribulations you have faced and explore how you might use your experiences to help others.

If you know your passion and mission, but cannot see the bridge from here to there–no worries, just start with one step; build one piece at a time.

If you are already fulfilling your mission in life, good for you.

Whatever you choose to do, when things get tough and people doubt your choices (fair warning, both will happen), remember:

> *It is not the critic who counts; not the man who points out how the strong man stumbles, or where the doer of deeds could have done them better. The credit belongs to the man who is actually in the arena, whose face is marred by dust and sweat and blood; who strives valiantly; who errs, who comes short again and again, because there is no effort without error and shortcoming; but who does actually strive to do the deeds; who knows great enthusiasms, the great devotions; who spends himself in a worthy cause; who at the best knows in the end the triumph of high achievement, and who at the worst, if he fails, at least fails while daring greatly, so that his place shall never be with those cold and timid souls who neither know victory nor defeat.*
>
> - Theodore Roosevelt

11

Lessons Learned

... but we rejoice in our sufferings,
knowing that suffering produces endurance,
and endurance produces character,
and character produces hope ...
Romans 5:3-4

It sounds so contradictory and cliché, but I am truly thankful for the trials through which I have come. The struggles I faced made me stronger, more mindful, and more empathetic toward others. If I had the chance to turn back time and relive my life in a way that meant avoiding all the sadness, heartache, anger, and pain; I wouldn't take it. I have learned so much about myself, about my marriage, about people, and about life in general.

If I could turn back time, what I would do is learn life's lessons more quickly. For that reason, I share in this chapter a few of the lessons I've learned along our journey in hopes that you will be able to avoid some of the mistakes I made, or at least learn the lessons more hastily than I did.

Some of the lessons seem simple at first glance. Some are thoughts we've all heard before, over and over–things

I *knew,* but had to learn how to *apply.* Other lessons were brand new to me and seemed to show up out of left field at just the right time.

Hopefully you will read this list and say, "I've been there and learned those. Wow, she really is a slow learner." However, if that is not your reaction, I hope my sharing helps you in some small way.

- I don't know anyone else's story. I cannot walk in anyone else's shoes. What I can do is interact with others from a place of love, compassion, and patience.
- I don't have to fix all my problems at once.
- There is no *right* way to deal with life's challenges, or even life's victories. My personality and life experiences make me as unique as my fingerprints.
- Occasional silence and solitude are golden.
- Busyness can mask as a shield for avoiding painful thoughts and emotions.
- Balance is key. Everything in moderation.
- I don't have to maintain the appearance that all is well all the time with everyone. It's okay to let my guard down.
- It is important to *feel* my feelings.

- It is important to *speak* my feelings.
- Chronic physical and emotional pain are *equally* traumatic.
- Intimacy and sex are not synonymous, but they are related.
- Sexuality isn't my womanhood.
- Love and intimacy can exist in a marriage even when sex is impossible.
- Love is more often an *action we choose* than a *feeling we feel.*
- I need support–especially when I think I don't.
- I can be real, open, and honest without telling everyone everything. It is okay to share my thoughts selectively.
- It is advantageous to have someone who will listen without judgment or attachment to the outcome. Sometimes that might be a friend, other times that might be a trained professional.
- "Hope is not an emotion;" it's a learned *cognitive process.*[1]
- You get what you pay for. Literally. High-quality care can be expensive, but it's usually worth the expense in the end.

- Sometimes the greatest consideration when comparing cost to benefit is the potential mental toll.

- Sometimes my best is simply showing up.

- Where was God during the hard times? He was there. Always. Patiently waiting.

- God never gave me more than I could handle. Close. But not quite.

- Life takes grit and a will to persevere.

- It is possible to turn anxiety into excitement.

- Perfection is a myth. Rather than aiming to be perfect, I will aim to be better today than yesterday.

- Comparison is the thief of joy. - *Thomas Jefferson*

I am thankful that I now live from a place of understanding and realization that I cannot know what anyone else is dealing with at any given moment. When it comes to our interaction with those whose paths cross ours, compassion is a must.

Could it be that the waitress who seems like a grouch has an abusive father or was recently widowed? Maybe the cashier at the grocery store who can't seem to get anything right as she rings up your groceries was just given the eviction notice she'd been dreading. Or possibly, like me, the friend who seems distant is dealing with a kind of pain he or she just isn't ready to share.

In short, the bottom line is this: Be kind. Just be kind. And listen. Be the person others know they can reveal their inner-most feelings to and simply let them speak about any and every topic. Then, if they need sympathy, give it. If they need silence, give that. If they need advice, give that too.

We would not have survived our journey through pain had it not been for the patience, kindness, and listening ears of family, friends, and most of my healthcare providers - even when none of them knew the extent to which we were suffering.

In addition, we certainly could not have been as strong as we (usually) were throughout this journey had it not been for our faith in God and our trust in His eternal plan. In all reality, we are only here for a short time. And while we may have to be tough while we're here (God never promised life would be easy) He gives us the assurance that He will provide peace and comfort to us during our lives on earth if we put our faith in Him.

Conclusion

Are you waiting to read our fairy tale's majestic ending? The point in the story where life returns to perfect bliss? The time when the screen reads, "And they lived happily ever after?"

Well, here it is. The real life version anyway. After 13 years, more than 20 healthcare providers, at least 30 treatment attempts, and too many financial expenditures to even attempt calculating, I am finally able to experience pain-free intercourse. More importantly, Alan and I learned to work through our differences and improve our communication skills to finally reach a level of comfortable intimacy. Granted, there is always room for improvement. Relationships are like every living thing–if they aren't growing, they are dying. But the fact that ours stopped dying and started growing is truly a reason to celebrate.

Words cannot express how thankful I am that we pressed on. That we searched until we found help and found the correct solutions. That we realized pain was not normal, and I found the voice to speak up (sadly, as many as 40 percent of women with sexual pain don't seek care[1]).

Like I said throughout the book, finding answers to heal my physical pain was extremely difficult. I wanted to ignore it. To forget about that part of our lives. It took me years to understand the importance of the sexual aspect of our relationship. But, as the authors of *When Sex Hurts* explain, "The thing is, no matter how much we try to minimize it's importance or focus on other aspects of a relationship, sex *is* a crucial part of a healthy relationship.[2]"

I am equally thankful that Alan and I both had the will, and found the strength from God, to work through the emotional struggles of a marriage lined with thorns. For those just beginning this journey, or who are still in the middle of it, trust me–the roses are worth it.

As I bring this book to a close, I sit humbled and grateful for the opportunity to share my journey and my thoughts with you. I don't know your story, or your motivation for learning about mine. What I do know is that we all have struggles, trials, and adversities, and I pray that something I wrote on these pages will help you in some way.

If you are a woman dealing with any sort of sexual pain, and it bothers you, please know that pain is not normal - it is a sign of dysfunction - and that you have a right to more than just duty sex. Help is available and I hope you will seek it.

I will leave you with one final, hopeful thought:

Hardships often prepare people
for an extraordinary destiny.
C.S. Lewis

Appendix A - Nutrition

Good nutrition creates health in all areas of our existence. All parts are interconnected.
T. Collin Campbell

As I mentioned in the book, I am passionate about nutrition and "alternative" medicine. I remain in awe of the body's innate ability to heal itself when given the proper fuel. I believe our diets have a direct affect on the way we feel, not only physically, but also mentally and spiritually. As an Integrative Nutrition Health Coach, one of my goals is to help others utilize the power of foods, and other healing tools God created for us, to live life to the fullest.

Because of my background, I nearly fainted when I reviewed the list of "suggested post-op foods" before my vestibulectomy. The foods listed were not healing foods, so I wanted to share some examples of the foods I chose instead.

SIMPLE POST-OP SELECTIONS

- Fresh fruits and vegetables - whole, blended, juiced, raw, steamed, roasted, mashed
- Broth-based soups and stews–loaded with vegetables, and a bit of lean red meat (great source of iron, Omega-3s, and B-vitamins to support healing)
- Sprouted grain toast, wild rice, nuts, seeds

- Hydration - Great choices include water (plain or infused), lemonade, green tea, and freshly-squeezed juices. Caution: Caffeine can be dehydrating and carbonation can lead to gas and bloating

NOTE ABOUT SUPPLEMENTS

Also in the book, I mentioned my use of food-based supplements and essential oils. While I am avid proponent of supplements, oils, homeopathic medicine, etc., it is important to know that all products are not created equal. Because they are not regulated by the FDA, it is important to do your own research to verify the quality and purity of supplements you purchase, and to ensure they are free of contaminants and fillers. United States Pharmacopeia (USP), NSF International (NSF), and ConsumerLab offer third-party testing and certification of products. Another great resource is the *Physicians' Desk Reference.*

For more information about these topics visit
www.thornsandroses.us

Appendix B – Practitioners

Great practitioners are out there. Search until you find one. Your pain is real and you deserve proper care.

GREAT PRACTITIONERS ...

- ✓ Hear what patients tell them
- ✓ Share concern for the issues that concern their patients
- ✓ Stay up-to-date on the latest medical research
- ✓ Recommend a holistic approach; treating body and mind
- ✓ Validate a patient's pain, even when they can't *see* a cause
- ✓ Acknowledge the big picture of intimacy in relationships
- ✓ Strive to educate patients and provide tools/resources
- ✓ Continue working until their patient is well

NOT SO GREAT PRACTITIONERS ...

- ⃠ Tell a patient it's all in his/her head
- ⃠ Refuse to refer patients to specialists
- ⃠ Discourage second opinions
- ⃠ Downplay the severity of one's pain and its affects on life
- ⃠ Become irritated when patients ask questions
- ⃠ Claim to have all the answers
- ⃠ Fail to consider a patient's history
- ⃠ Tell patients to ignore the pain
- ⃠ Merely treat symptoms and neglect making a diagnosis
- ⃠ Recommend an extra glass of wine as a cure
- ⃠ Say there is no solution; give up on patients

Resources

Tulsa Women's Health Alliance
www.tulsawomenshealthalliance.com

National Vulvodynia Association
www.nva.org

National Association of Nurse Practitioners in Women's Health
www.npwh.org

International Society for the Study of Women's Sexual Health
www.isswsh.org

Institute for Sexual Medicine
www.sexualmed.org

American Association of Sexuality Educators, Counselors and Therapists
www.aasect.org

National Association of Cognitive Behavioral Therapists
www.nacbt.org

Association of Behavioral and Cognitive Therapies
www.abct.org

Academy of Cognitive Therapy
www.academyofct.org

American Physical Therapy Association
www.womenshealthapta.org

EMDR International Association
www.emdria.site-ym.com

Dr. Irwin Goldstein
San Diego Sexual Medicine
www.sandiegosexualmedicine.com
For a free phone consultation call - 619-265-8865

Dr. Corey Babb
Oklahoma State University Center for Women's Sexual Health
https://www.facebook.com/DrCoreyBabb/
918-586-4500

When Sex Hurts - Goldstein, Goldstein & Pukall
When Sex Isn't Good - Arleque & Goldstein
The Vulvodynia Survival Guide - Glazer & Rodke
The V Book - Stewart
Start Talking: Intimacy - Hague & Smith
Intended for Pleasure - Wheat
Daring Greatly - Brown
The Gifts of Imperfection - Brown
Breaking the Habit of Being Yourself - Dispenza
Feelings Buried Alive Never Die - Truman
Invitation to Solitude & Silence - Barton
Your Body Speaks Your Mind - Shapiro

VagiKool
www.vagikool.com

End Notes

Preface

1. Brown, Brene. *Daring Greatly: How the Courage to Be Vulnerable Transforms the Way We Live, Love, Parent, and Lead.* S.l.: Avery Publishing Group, 2015. p. 32

Chapter 1

1. Hillock, David , and Mike Schnelle. *Roses in Oklahoma.* PDF. Stillwater: Oklahoma Cooperative Extension Service.
2. Wheat, Ed, and Gaye Wheat. *Intended for pleasure: sex technique and sexusal fulfillment in Christian marriage.* 4th ed. Grand Rapids, MI: Revell, 2010. p. 33
3. Goldstein, Andrew, Caroline F. Pukall, and Irwin Goldstein. *When sex hurts: a womans guide to banishing sexual pain.* Cambridge, Mass: Da Capo Lifelong,
   2011. p. 52

Chapter 3

1. "Vaginal Septum." Advanced Reproductive Medicine - University of Colorado. Accessed November 4, 2017. https://arm.coloradowomens health.com/info/reproductive-disorders/vaginal-septum.

Chapter 4

1. Smith, Y. R. "Pronociceptive and Antinociceptive Effects of Estradiol through Endogenous Opioid Neurotransmission in Women." *Journal of Neuroscience* 26, no. 21 (2006): 5777-785. doi:10.1523/jneurosci.5223-05.2006.
2. Sofronescu, Alina G. "Estradiol." Medscape. March 18, 2015. https://emedicine.medscape.com/article/2089003-overview.
3. "What are vaginal dilators?" International Society for Sexual Medicine. Accessed November 17, 2017. http://www.issm.info/sexual-health-qa/what-are-vaginal-dilators/.

4. "Biofeedback." Pelvic Floor Center. Accessed November 26, 2017. http://www.pelvicfloorcenter.org/content/biofeedback.
5. "The dangers of long-term and continuous use of topical steroids." Health24. July 9, 2014. Accessed November 24, 2017. http://www.health24.com/Medical/Skin/Health-tips/The-dangers-of-long-term-and-continuous-use-of-topical-steroids-20140530.
6. "Pudendal Peripheral Nerve Block." JLR Center for Pain Medicine. Accessed November 26, 2017. http://www.centerforpain.com/treatments/neuropathic-pain/pudendal-peripheral-nerve-block.
7. Goldstein, Goldstein, & Pukall, 184-185.
8. Glazer, Howard I., and Gae Rodke. *The vulvodynia survival guide.* Oakland, CA: New Harbinger, 2002. p. 10.

Chapter 5

1. Goldstein, Andrew T. "Cotton Swab Test." Sex in the 21st Century. Accessed November 20, 2017. https://sexualmed.org/diagnostic-tests/cotton-swab-test/.
2. "Vestibulectomy." Sex in the 21st Century. Accessed November 20, 2017. https://sexualmed.org/treatments/vestibulectomy/.

Chapter 6

1. Henzell, Helen, Karen Berzins, and Jennifer Langford. "Provoked Vestibulodynia: Current Perspectives." *International Journal of Women's Health* 9 (September 11, 2017): 631-42. doi:10.2147/IJWH.S113416.
2. "Key Statistics from the National Survey of Family Growth - C Listing." National Survey of Family Growth. https://www.cdc.gov/nchs/nsfg/key_statistics/c.htm#contraception.

Chapter 8

1. Goetsch, MF. "Incidence of Bartholin's duct occlusion after superficial localized vestibulectomy." *American Journal of Obstetrics and Gynecology,* June 2009. Accessed November 1, 2017. doi:10.1016/j.ajog.2009.02.037.
2. "Bartholin's Cyst." Mayo Clinic. https://www.mayoclinic.org/diseases-conditions/bartholin-cyst/basics/definition/con-20026333.
3. "Marsupialization." Wikipedia. Accessed November 26, 2017. https://en.wikipedia.org/wiki/Marsupialization.

Chapter 9

1. Brown, 137.
2. Burton, Neel. "Our Hierarchy of Needs." Psychology Today. May 23, 2012. https://www.psychologytoday.com/blog/hide-and-seek/201205/our-hierarchy-needs.
3. Hanscom, David. *Back in control: a surgeons roadmap out of chronic pain.* Seattle, WA: Vertus Press, 2017. p. 90
4. Handel, Steven. "Classification of Emotions." The Emotion Machine. May 24, 2011. Accessed November 6, 2017. http://www.theemotion machine.com/classification-of-emotions/.
5. Goldstein, Goldstein, and Pukall. p. 59.
6. Hanscom, 92.
7. Nagoski, Emily. *Come as you are: the surprising new science that will transform your sex life*. New York: Simon & Schuster Paperbacks, 2015. p. 317.
8. Truman, Karol. *Feelings Buried Alive Never Die*. St. George: Olympus Distributing, 2003. p. 5.
9. Hanscom, 116.
10. Dispenza, Joe. *Breaking the Habit of Being Yourself.* Hay House, 2012. p. 61-63.
11. Ibid., 69.
12. Hanscom, 116.
13. Wheat, 23.
14. Dispenza, 4.
15. Shapiro, Deb. *Your Body Speaks Your Mind*. Sounds True, 2006. p. 14.

Figure 9.1 created by J. Finkelstein https://commons.wikimedia.org/wiki/File:Maslow%27s_hierarchy_of_needs.svg
Figure 9.2 http://friedtechnology.blogspot.com/2015/11/use-this-feelings-wheel-by-kaitlin-robb.html
Figure 9.3 created by J. Cole

Chapter 10

1. Cohen, Elizabeth. "'Female Viagra' Gets Mixed Reviews." CNN Health. March 1, 2016. http://www.cnn.com/2016/02/29/health/female-viagra-gets-mixed-reviews/index.html.

Chapter 11

1. Brown, 239.

Conclusion

1. Goldstein, Goldstein, & Pukall, 4.
2. Goldstein, Goldstein, & Pukall, 52.

Acknowledgments

First, to my remarkable husband, better half, and soulmate. You are the kindest, most patient person I have ever known. Thank you for knowing how to handle my "crazy" and being my pillar of strength and safety. Words cannot express the love and appreciation I have for you. Love you more.

To my three amazing children–my blessings from God. Thank you for motivating me to be my best so I can teach you to be your best.

To Irwin ("Dr. G") and Sue Goldstein who went above and beyond to give me the strength and courage to become pain-free and share my heart with the world. You became family along our journey, and we are immensely blessed to know you.

To Corey Babb, D.O., for your willingness to put together an incredible chapter for this book, even when I didn't give you much time to make that happen. And more importantly for creating an environment in Oklahoma to compassionately and comfortably treat women with sexual dysfunction. You are an answer to many, many prayers.

To Susan Bachmann, LPC; Chad Edwards, D.O.; and Dannelle Newnam, LPC, for your expert contributions to this book. And more importantly, for your expert contributions to my life.

To my friend and co-dreamer Megan Warner. What would I do without you helping me put my big plans into action and enthusiastically listening to all my wild ideas? Above all else, thank you for your brutal honesty when I need it. I owe you an açaí bowl.

To Laura, Erin, & Nicki, for being open and honest about your struggles and for your three years of consistently encouraging me to make both the support group and this book happen.

To Traci Owen, for sharing my grand vision. I am excited to see where God leads us, friend.

To Becky Wilcox, for being a "yes" woman anytime anything is needed for the TWHA. And for being an amazing PT.

To the providers of the Tulsa Women's Health Alliance: Karol Andrew, Dr. Corey Babb, Susan Bachmann, Dr. Chad Edwards, Whitney Ellsworth, Dr. Irwin Goldstein, Jessica Kanwhen, Amanda Killian, Emma Strande, Megan Warner, Becky Wilcox and Summer Wyers. I am still amazed at how quickly our special group came together. Thank you for all you do to support women and for your understanding and patience as I went a bit MIA for a few months to make this book happen.

To the staff of San Diego Sexual Medicine and the staff of the National Vulvodynia Association, I sincerely appreciate the unwavering support and research you have provided for me and for all women walking in similar shoes.

To all those who encouraged me in this process and graciously helped edit this work.

Finally, to the Institute for Integrative Nutrition for offering the "Launch Your Dream Book" course at the perfect time in my life. The course modules and ongoing, bio-individual support gave me the passion and drive to get the words out of my head and onto these pages.

About the Author

J. Cole is a passionate advocate for women's health, serving as a support leader for the National Vulvodynia Association. In 2016, she organized the Tulsa Women's Health Alliance–a group of healthcare providers in and around Tulsa, Oklahoma, who strive to educate, support, and empower women with pelvic pain. Cole is also an Integrative Nutrition Health Coach and founder of Fundamentally Well. Cole enjoys decorating, practicing yoga, having friends in her home, and being horseback. Her favorite things include crème brûlée, October in Oklahoma, San Diego, fresh watermelon, açaí bowls, long-sleeve t-shirts and mornings spent on the porch with her Bible, a warm drink, a cool breeze, and the sound of cows grazing on green grass. Cole lives in Oklahoma with her husband and their children.

www.thornsandroses.us
thornsandrosesbook@gmail.com
www.fundamentallywell.com